THE REHAB WEIGHT LOSS PLAN

SHAUN WRIGHT

The Rehab Weight Loss Book was written Shaun Wright

ISBN: 9798666133996

Further information can be obtained from:

www.rehab-weight loss-plan.com

Contents

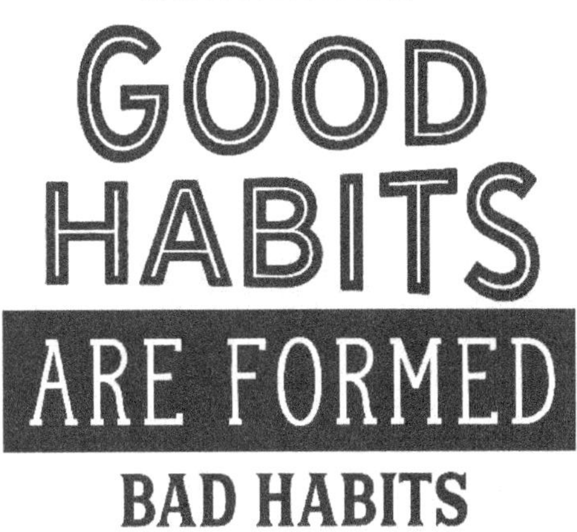

GOOD
HABITS
ARE FORMED
BAD HABITS
WE FALL INTO

1. INTRODUCTION

When it comes to eating food, I am the same as any other person on this planet. I eat too much, go on the latest diet, get bored, then back to my normal diet and the foods that I crave. I live in this constant 'weight on, weight off, weigh on' cycle resulting in my weight going up and down like a yo-yo. One of the wonders of the world is why it takes four to five weeks for me to remove the weight that I so easily put on in two to three days, whilst on a weekend break? I have given up the dream of having 'hips like a racing snake'.

Over the years, I have tried several different diets, such as Atkins and Weight Watchers, with varying success. These weight loss plans come up with credible facts and figures as to why we should be on their recommended diet. They offer hope for most of us when we are in a desperate state of mind. However, in most cases, these diets are short term fixes and not long-term solutions to help us maintain our ideal body weight.

I find that their recommended diets completely miss the point and they never address the fundamental reason why we always fail when dieting, even though our intentions are good. Our daily motivation, attitude, rationale for justifying our food intake is hugely influenced by our subconscious minds, which have been created and manipulated by our parents throughout our childhood. We were constantly programmed that 'more is good' and we now have set beliefs that influence our rationale for our food choices. The main reason why most diets fail is that they only highlight the dieting method (e.g. how to reduce our calories or carbohydrates) without addressing our current eating habits. These are well-established habits, we eat like we have always eaten, on autopilot, and this is our main barrier to implementing a successful weight loss programme.

Furthermore, for most of us, we have never quantified what our current daily food consumption is. The result is that we are constantly eating larger food portions than we need, even though it does not necessarily mean we are enjoying it more. If we don't know how much food we are consuming, then we will never know how much to reduce our intake by to lose weight. We have never been told how much food is enough to maintain our ideal weight and for most of our lives, our food portion sizes have been determined by others, such as our parents or third-parties (e.g. fast food outlets).

Unless we address these two underlying issues, by focusing on the rationale for our eating habits and food choices, by becoming more aware of our food intake, we will be constantly on this 'weight on, weight off, weigh on' cycle, experiencing further dieting failures. Our weight loss plan also needs to be as simple as possible, as we do not want to spend all our time counting calories or working out the carbohydrate or fat content in our foods.

The underlying message of this book is that we need to treat our body like an engine. An engine is a mechanical 'thing' that is not influenced by our subconscious mind, our upbringing, or the latest supermarket sales offers. We need to consider food as a fuel, a unit of energy, which needs to be constantly monitored and adjusted, ensuring that our engine is consuming what is only necessary. The future success of your weight loss plan will depend on how successful you are in managing to disconnect your subconscious mind from your daily food intake, the fuel that you are supplying to your engine.

If you have been frequently experiencing dieting failures, and you are looking for underlying reasons, the Rehab Weight Loss Plan will provide these answers for you.

The Rehab Weight Loss Plan consists of a simple five-step management plan, developed using common sense. We are highlighting the importance of having to first, change your eating habits, then introduce a formal, structured weight loss management plan.

A summary of do's and don'ts whilst on the Rehab Weight Loss Plan:

- We can eat and enjoy our favourite foods
- There is no counting of calories
- There is no counting of carbohydrate or fat content
- There is no suggested fitness regime
- There are no recommended recipes in this book
- There is no self-promotion section highlighting or selling the latest dietary products (e.g. protein drinks and snacks)

The Rehab Weight Loss Plan will help you:

- Understand how the subconscious mind influences your current eating habits, the rationale for your food intake
- Help you to re-programme (rehab) your subconscious mind to ensure that old eating habits don't dictate your food intake
- Make you more aware of your current food consumption, and how to reduce daily intake
- Implement a simple food consumption reduction plan to help you achieve your weight loss goals
- Improve your overall wellbeing

You will need the following to successfully implement the Rehab Weight Loss Plan:

- Acknowledge that you need to change your eating habits as they are sabotaging your good dieting intentions
- The ability to count to at least 50 at any one time
- A desire to lose weight and have a degree of self-control to stay on the simple five-step plan

For most of us, this is a small sacrifice, especially when we know that the benefits of losing weight far surpass those of being overweight. Furthermore, changing our eating habits won't cost us money to implement.

The book will help reconnect to the joys of eating food, as every meal we have should be a pleasant, memorable experience.

2. BACKGROUND – FOOD FOR THOUGHT

At any one time, it is estimated that 60% (estimated 40 million people), in the UK population are on a diet and signed up to the 'weight on, weight off, weight on' cycle. [1] For most of us who have previously been on a diet, we can confirm that it is a constant challenge to find a diet that works, one that helps us first lose weight and then maintain our ideal weight. Why is it that even when we have the best of intentions, dieting is so difficult and a constant challenge?

We have a huge global problem called obesity, with it the associated long-term health problems and treatment costs. So, let's look at the bigger picture and confirm some facts.

- **World obesity:** Data from the World Obesity Federation (WOF) show that worldwide obesity has tripled since 1975. In 2016, an estimated 1.9 billion adults (39%) were overweight, of these, 650 million (13%) were obese. [2] Obesity is continuing to increase, and it is predicted that one-fifth (20%) of all adults (approx. 2.7 billion) worldwide will be overweight or obese by 2025, many of whom are likely to end up needing additional medical care. [3]

- **Deaths related to bad diet:** Research has confirmed that poor diet, eating too much processed foods and sugary drinks, were responsible for more deaths (e.g. Cardiovascular disease and type-2 diabetes) than any other risk group (e.g. smoking). The study found that poor diet was responsible for at least 11 million deaths in 2017, representing 22% of all global deaths. [4] Other long-term illnesses associated with poor diet include insulin resistance, musculoskeletal disorders (osteoarthritis), some cancers, and a range of physical disabilities.

- **Childhood obesity:** Over 340 million children and adolescents, aged 5 to 19, were considered overweight or obese in 2016. The number of overweight or childhood obese infants (0 to 5 years) was 40 million in 2018. [5] It is estimated that by 2030, 250 million children will be considered obese. [6]

- **Cost of poor health:** The cost of treating poor health, caused by obesity around the world, will top an estimated $1.2tn every year, from 2025. Unless more is more done to prevent the rapidly worsening epidemic, countries are looking at a very steep rise in costs that we, the taxpayers, will have to pay. [7]

- **Low-income countries:** In low-income countries or regions (e.g. Africa), the obesity rate among children and adults has increased significantly in recent years. Low-income countries that have inadequate healthcare systems, and barely manage to cope with local infectious diseases, have neither the money nor staff to deal with the epidemic of chronic illness associated with obesity. [8]

These above facts are staggering, to say the least and how did we get to this point?

Over the past 50 years, human beings have not significantly grown any bigger in genetic make-up or physical stature, in overall height or build. To break it down in simpler terms, our mouths and stomachs are the same sizes as they have ever been.

It is a well-documented fact that our parents, and grandparents, worked harder than our generation as there was more manual labour. They may have worked in a factory, which was labour intensive, with limited time for socializing and relaxing. There was less public transport and most daily chores (e.g. washing clothes) required more physical effort and there were extra everyday activities (e.g. walking).

With the invention of computers, the world has become a more automated place and machines are doing the work that was previously done by manual labour. Our automobiles and public transport systems have improved to a point where we prefer to use these rather than walking. Furthermore, with the invention of computer games, our children don't have to leave the comfort of their room to get mentally stimulated. Although this is convenient for most of us, it does mean that we are exercising far less and is one of the main factors for us being overweight.

Modern diets

There has never been a time in the history of mankind where most people have an abundance of good, high-quality nutritious food that can be conveniently purchased locally. If we wanted, we can now order the latest low-carb, no-fat meal and get it delivered to our doorstep. We have the spare time to join a local gym, have a swim or go for a walk in the park.

Governments have, over the years, spent millions promoting healthy eating and they have implemented nationwide dietary campaigns, encouraging us to be more mindful of the types of foods we are consuming. When it comes to nutrition, we are now more educated and food aware, compared to our parents. We endeavour to avoid the consumption of processed foods loaded with calories, carbohydrates, sugar or, trans fats. We all know that poor eating habits lead to obesity, resulting in poor health and premature death, all preventable through the intervention of a well-balanced diet.

However, these messages don't appear to be working. Do we give up and accept that worldwide obesity is now a fact of life and that we have limited control of the situation? As we are the ones who were responsible for putting us in this place in the first instance, there should be no reason why we can't reverse this growing trend.

Looking at the bigger picture, there are certain population groups, and members of our society, who are less affected by obesity. If we could understand why they are not affected, then this could help us come up with a solution to reduce obesity.

Population groups and individuals less affected by obesity

We should remind ourselves that obesity doesn't appear to affect certain population groups or members of our society, namely:

- **Africans in rural Africa:** Whilst driving through rural Africa, you will rarely see someone who is overweight. Their income can be as low as $1.25 a day. [9] They live off maize, vegetables and fruits that are freely available off the nearest tree. They are 'skinny' as their consumption, mouthfuls of food is far less than the average Western European. In the worldwide league table of the countries with the worst obesity rates, there is not one African country in the top 35 countries. [10]

- **Homeless people:** It is generally accepted that most homeless people are not overweight, due to unfortunate social and economic circumstances forced on them. This is not due to what type of food they eat. They will eat whatever food that is placed in front of them, or what they can rummage through in the nearest fast food rubbish bin. The reason they are not overweight is because of their lack of food, the reduced food intake going into their mouths daily. They are also not influenced by the latest supermarket or fast food sales offers.

- **POWs (prisoners of war):** We always associate POWs as being excessively 'slim' in body weight due to the absence of food. They were not able to choose what food, or how much they wanted to eat and most, unfortunately, starved to death.

- **Italian diets:** There are several nationalities that have a heavy carbohydrate based daily diet. It is generally accepted that Italian children will eat more pasta and pizza during their lifetime, compared with most kids around the world. These foods are recognised as the nation's favourite dishes and are consumed daily. In the worldwide league table of the countries with the worst obesity rates, Italy is not in the top 50 countries. [11] This suggests that high-carbohydrate diets are okay in moderation.

The above facts clearly highlight that it is not what we eat but how much we consume that is key. Yes, we should all be eating foods that are healthy, high in protein, and nutrients. However, if we are not controlling the amount entering our bodies, we will gain weight and have obesity issues.

There is no social or economic class discrimination when it comes to obesity. People who are fortunate to have upper or middle-class financial incomes are just as overweight as those on a lower income. We typically associate those, in the low-income band, to regularly eat high-carbohydrate, processed meals. In fact, the more money we have, the more opportunities there are to be overweight. Overindulging on lobster, in a Thermidor sauce meal, is the same as eating a cheap, large pizza. If you are eating more food than your body needs, you will be exceeding your daily recommended allowance and you will ultimately gain weight.

It is obviously clear, from the above facts, that if we want to lose weight, we need to reduce our daily food consumption, the number of mouthfuls going into our bodies. This will result in fewer calories having to be processed. If we are constantly eating less than we did yesterday, or less this week than we did last week, there is no reason why we should not lose weight. If this is so simple, then why can't we readily lose weight and why do our diets always fail?

The obvious answer is that our good dieting intentions are constantly been sabotaged by our poor eating habits and food choices, that we have adopted from our childhood. Our established habits have been 'telling' us when we are hungry and what we should eat.

These underlying habits determine our motivation, attitude or rationale for our daily food intake and are influenced by both, personal (e.g. childhood and psychological) and external (e.g. social and environmental) factors. Furthermore, a large part of our daily food consumption is determined by third parties, such as supermarkets and restaurants, resulting in us having limited control of our daily food intake.

If we are wanting to stop this 'weight on, weight off, weight on' dieting cycle, we must first address, and then alter, our eating habits before we implement our latest recommended diet. Once we have introduced our new, good eating habits to our daily lives, this will help us stay on our diets and achieve our weight loss goals.

3. THE REHAB WEIGHT LOSS PLAN OVERVIEW

Introduction

Some definitions that we need to be aware of:

'Rehab' is short for rehabilitation and is defined as any process designed to help a person recover from a threat to their wellbeing (e.g. illness or addiction).

'Eating habits' is defined as how people eat (e.g. their motivation, attitude, and rationale) and include their food choice (i.e. the type of food that they eat). The source of our habits comes from our long-established beliefs. These beliefs influence our eating habits (i.e. we need to eat three meals daily) and our food choices (i.e. bigger is better).

'Beliefs' is defined as an acceptance that something exists or is true, especially something without proof. Our beliefs are influenced by our childhood, past experiences, social environment (media), and our knowledge at the time.

Our well-established beliefs and habits, the rationale of why we eat, play a significant role in our daily food consumption. However, they have no association with us being hungry. We are overweight because we have let our eating habits tell us when we are hungry. On the Rehab Weight Loss Plan, our main objective is to challenge our existing beliefs and 'rehab' our eating habits.

To replace these poor habits, with good ones, we need to first change any negative, underlying beliefs that we have. In short, if there is no 'rehab' of our existing beliefs and eating habits, then there is a good chance that we will experience another dieting failure.

Signing-up to the Rehab Weight Loss Plan should be considered as a necessary life-changing process, a habit-changing strategy designed to improve our thought processes (i.e. our eating habits) to ensure that they don't influence our food consumption. We could say that the book is a habit-changing diet, rather than one promoting a dieting method (e.g.

eating low-carb foods).

The main barrier for most of us is that our eating habits are 'invisible', we are not aware of them until they are pointed out to us. Once we are aware that they exist, we can then introduce a habit-changing strategy so that our old habits don't dictate our food intake. With our new 'less is good' habits in place, we only then introduce our weight loss management plan.

Our old eating habits have, over a period, caused us to regularly overeat and we are now overweight. Once we have successfully implemented our 'less is good' eating habits, they become well-established, we will automatically start losing weight. We won't have to 'sign-up' to the latest 'fad' diet or purchase another low-carb recipe book.

The five-step Rehab Weight Loss Plan overview

To successfully implement a project, say in a commercial environment, we need to have a structured management plan in place, highlighting every step of the way to implementation. Typically, the management plan would comprise a well-established five-step process and include the following:

Identify the issue (step 1),
Carrying out a period of monitoring (step 2),
Implement a management plan for improvement (step 3),
Evaluate the performance (step 4),
Manage the plan going forward (step 5).

The Rehab Weight Loss Plan includes all the above principles, plus some small changes. The process consists of a three-stage, five-step plan, as highlighted below:

Stage 1: Review and rehab our eating habits
- **Step 1: Understand our eating habits**. We address our current beliefs and eating habits, our rationale for our food consumption and why our diets fail. We explore the role that our subconscious mind plays in our food habits (e.g. why we eat in autopilot), and how third parties influence our rationale when it comes to food choice.
- **Step 2: Rehab our eating habits**. Now that we are aware of our eating habits, we then 'rehab' these so that our rationale for our food intake is not in subconscious mode.

10

Stage 2: Implement the Rehab Weight Loss Plan

- **Step 3: Create our food consumption baseline and set reduction targets.** We create our food consumption baseline, so that we know what our current daily consumption is. With this information, we can now set our mouthful reduction targets to achieve our weight loss goals.
- **Step 4: Implement the Rehab Weight Loss Plan.** Knowing what our daily consumption is, we can now implement our weight loss plan which consists of reducing the overall volume of our daily food consumption.

Stage 3: Improve our food choice habits

- **Step 5: Rehab our food choice habits.** Having implemented our weight loss plan, we can now review and improve our food choice habits (e.g. when preparing meals or in a restaurant).

Implementation of the Rehab Weight Loss Plan

Typically, we would expect to see changes in our eating habits, and signs of weight loss, from week two onwards. Whilst on the Rehab Weight Loss Plan, if you lose your way, you can refer to the below flow process illustration to give you an idea of what stage you are at.

Overview of The Rehab Weight Loss Plan [12]

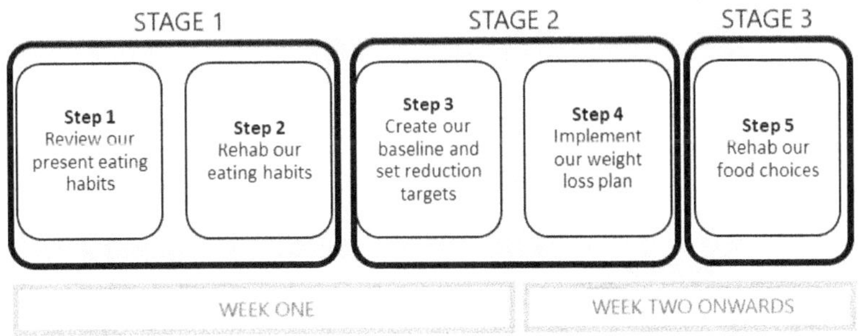

4. WHY MOST DIETS FAIL (Step 1)

Step one of The Rehab Weight Loss Plan:

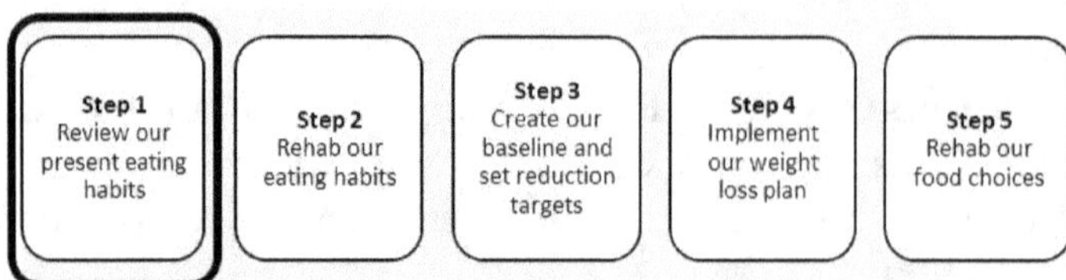

A considerable amount of research has been done of why most common diets fail and there is a range of psychological factors that play a part. Understanding what part these factors play when we are on a diet will give us an indication of where we are going wrong.

Below are some of the common reasons why we fail to stay on a planned diet and how The Rehab Weight Loss Plan will help us overcome these issues:

We are not aware of why our previous diets failed

Unless we have an understanding why our previous diets have failed, there is a good possibility that we will fail on our next diet. We need to know what the underlying causes are; why, when and where our dieting failures are happening.

Most diets recommend that we control, or restrict our food intake, into our bodies. There is no reason, if we stay on their plan, why they should fail. In most cases, dieters have short term weight loss, however, with time they then tend to go back to their 'old ways', resulting in weight gain and another dieting failure.

Starting a new diet means we are clashing with our well-established eating habits that have been dictating our daily food consumption. The underlying issue here is not the implementation of the dieting method. Our dieting failures are due to existing beliefs, poor eating habits and food choices that we have adopted. We eat like we have always eaten and any major changes to our food intake on our new diet will be resisted, especially if we don't see any visible weight loss.

The Rehab Weight Loss Plan goes into detail as to what factors could possibly be harming our good dieting intentions and then provide simple habit-changing strategies to help us overcome these obstacles.

We are not aware of our daily food intake

Research has shown that a third of all people in the UK (an estimated 22 million) don't know how many calories they consume on an average day. [13] Even though governments have spent millions of pounds making us more food aware, yet we still appear to have limited understanding of what we need to do to lose weight.

As food portions vary in size, shape and calorie content, this makes it difficult to understand. If we have no idea what our food consumption is, how many calories we are consuming, how do we know how much to reduce by to lose weight?

Out of desperation, we attach ourselves to the latest dieting craze, hoping that this will be the answer to our prayers. However, most diets don't address what our current food consumption is and only highlight the method (e.g. eat low-carb meals).

The Rehab Weight Loss Plan consists of a formal, structured five-step plan to guide us through each step, ensuring that we are always in control. The plan addresses our current food consumption, by calculating our baseline food consumption. Once we have this information, we can put into place a simple food consumption reduction targets to reduce our daily intake.

Forbidden foods are more tempting

Most diets often involve quitting our favourite foods to help reduce our calorie intake. Giving up our favourite foods is not an easy process as our well-established habits will not disappear overnight. [14] Having had a simple violation of our chosen dieting rules, there will be a tendency to do it again, and again, as we start believing that we are not breaking the rules.

These forbidden foods, these treats, are habits that we have adopted, and this is one of the main reasons why modern diets fail. Any major changes to our eating habits will potentially result in another dieting failure.

In the first stages of the Rehab Weight Loss Plan, we can continue eating our regular meals so that we are not deprived of our favourite temptations.

Keep it simple stupid (KISS)

Most diets fail because they are too complicated to implement. If a task is too complicated and tedious, people have the tendency to lose interest and get bored quickly. For example, if we are counting calories, on a typical day we may have to add the following;

breakfast (450 kcal) + morning snack (75 kcal) + lunch (850 kcal) + afternoon cake (105 kcal) + supper (700 kcal) + drinks (500 kcal) + bedtime snack (65 kcal) = 2745 kcal for the day.

Trying to keep on track of our food consumption now becomes complicated and we will soon lose interest.

Furthermore, when counting calories, a trip to a restaurant becomes a nightmare, as we have no control over the portions that is served to us. The more add-ons to the plate, the more difficult it is to calculate the total calories.

On the Rehab Weight Loss Plan, we count the number of mouthfuls of food entering our body. A mouthful of food entering our mouth is, in most cases, a fixed volume (amount). For example;

breakfast (30 mouthfuls) + lunch (30 mouthfuls) + afternoon snack (5 mouthfuls) + supper (40 mouthfuls) = 105 mouthfuls for the day.

For most of us, to determine what our final food intake total was for the day, this can easily be calculated in our mind or recorded on a piece of paper. As we have all learnt to do simple counting exercises at school, monitoring our mouthfuls should be a simple procedure.

What can be simpler than appreciating how many mouthfuls you are currently eating, then knowing how much you need to reduce by over the coming weeks?

Summary:

- We need to understand why our diets fail
- Most of us are not aware how many calories we consume
- Modern diets can be complicated and rigorous
- We need to calculate our current daily food intake
- Modern diets involve giving up forbidden foods which may be a challenge

5. THE SUBCONSCIOUS MIND AND OUR FOOD INTAKE (Step 1)

Introduction

I am not a guru when it comes to understanding psychology and I am not going to pretend that I am. I have read extensively about psychology (the study of the mind and behaviour) and it is a fascinating subject. Extensive research has shown that our subconscious mind significantly influences every aspect of our daily life and that includes our daily food intake. [15]

Before we start our weight loss programme, we need to have a better understanding of how our everyday habits influence our food intake. Once we realise that these exist, we can then reprogram our subconscious minds, 'rehab' our eating habits, so our rationale to food consumption can be changed forever.

Old habits are hard to break

In simple terms, our brain operates either in conscious or subconscious mode. [16] During the day, we drift between our conscious and subconscious mind, depending on the circumstances at the time. When we are in a conscious mode, we are aware of what we are doing, working out what needs to be done, and how. We determine the solutions for making the right decisions and calculate the potential risks, making sure that our health and safety, or our security, are not compromised.

When in subconscious mode, we don't think about those minor, everyday decisions or actions because they happen automatically, as we have constantly repeated the same procedure. Simple 'things' that we do every day, such as driving, working, shopping, cooking and eating are done most of the time through habit, completely instinctively, on autopilot. [17] Our brain operates in the subconscious mode most of the time, typically making thousands of decisions in autopilot.

When we were children, we had no pre-existing beliefs or habits, we simply accepted that all the information we received, during our early childhood, was true. Our parents, teachers and those in authority, played a massive part in our upbringing, shaping our beliefs, habits and behaviour.

By the time we were 10 years old, we already had a solid foundation of beliefs and habits based on all that programming from those closest to us. Furthermore, our social environmental and external influences, such as media (television) that we were exposed to, also played a large role. With every experience, our subconscious mind was absorbing this information like a hard drive in a computer waiting to be used sometime in the future.

We often experienced a sense of guilt, or shame, if we did not fulfil the wishes of our parents or live up to their expectations. During our childhood, we learned to control our behaviour and thoughts, developing methods of coping with any negative input, especially if there was a form of reward associated with our good behaviour.

Some of our 'bad' habits that we have adopted include; overeating, smoking, excess alcohol consumption, drug addiction and watching pornography. We were not born with these habits and are all self-inflicted, often created in our childhood. Our established habits influence most aspects of our daily lives.

'Feel good' moments

Our subconscious mind is full of our past experiences, which include our 'feel good' moments. When we are in this mode, the day-to-day stress and strains of modern life disappear, and the world becomes a wonderful place again. Most of our 'feel good' moments occurred when we were in a secure, happy environment and generally linked with eating and family occasions.

For example, when we are in a restaurant, we habitually have a dessert. As we have just had a starter and a main course, this suggests that this additional add-on meal was not necessary as we could not possibly still be hungry. Or, having a chocolate bar as a treat, and accepting that we are not hungry, we are only eating this indulgence out of habit.

Eating desserts and chocolate bars have nothing to do with hunger, however, as we always enjoyed the treat, we will eat them out of habit. These are 'feel good' moments and no diet is going to stop us from having our favourite treat.

Well-established beliefs

New habits can be created in an instant, especially if there is a risk to our security or wellbeing. For example, when we buy a new car, we have a range of operational 'things' to understand and we have new procedures to adopt. However, within hours, they then become a regular habit.

If we know that our well-established habits are causing our dieting failures, why can't we instantly change our habits, so that we eat less? The reason is that our habits originate from our lifelong beliefs. We were not born with beliefs or habits. Through constant programming, starting in our childhood, our beliefs are formed, whether factual or not. [18] Our eating habits and food choices were created and supported by our underlying beliefs.

For example, if our parents had told us that chocolate has a high nutritional content and was good for us, we would not have thought about checking the nutritional data on the packaging, as this fact came from our parents. This belief would have stayed with us forever, well, until we were told otherwise.

Other 'real' examples of beliefs and habits that have stayed with us for most of our lives include; we always have layers of butter on our slices of bread, or we have always had a few teaspoons of sugar with tea. These habits have come from our childhood, from our parents. If they always put teaspoons of sugar in their cup of tea, then we just accepted that it was the norm.

If our parents allowed us to have an extra serving of cereal every morning, as they believed that cereal was good for you, then this habit would have lived with us for most of our lives. We all now know that certain cereal types, such as 'Frosted flakes', have excessive calories and sugar content, and we tend to avoid these cereals that we had as children.

If our parents used statements such as 'you eat like your father', or 'you are always hungry', these became beliefs and would have shaped our rationale for food for life and provide justification for eating more than we should be. Our diets fail because of our new habits (e.g. low-carb eating) clash with our well-established beliefs that caused our eating habits.

The main culprit, so to speak, was that we were led to believe that any information that our parents gave us was genuine fact and that 'more is good' when it came to food portion sizes. It was okay to ask for more, have another portion of food. Our parents may have justified our overindulgence with an excuse, 'he is a growing child'.

These well-established beliefs can be changed, especially if the new ones are factual and they make sense. We are all now adults and we can make our own rational decisions and create our own new beliefs, which will then become good habits.

Our food habits are on constant autopilot

Our subconscious process system, when it comes to our rationale for eating, is based on beliefs, habits and 'feel good' moments. [19] Our eating habits, whether good or bad, are mostly shaped through childhood experiences and often persist into adulthood. On most days, we eat on autopilot as we have eaten the same meal on hundreds of occasions. We tend to eat the way we have always done. In most cases, our food intake may have nothing to do with us being hungry.

We need to appreciate that there is no correlation between our eating habits and being hungry. Furthermore, certain beliefs that influenced our rationale for eating are not correct. Yet, for most of us, our habits and beliefs have been influencing our daily food consumption for most of our lives.

For example, when we miss a meal, for some reason, we don't then make up the difference by having an extra meal later in the day. Or, if we decide to miss one meal per day, say breakfast, after a few days it would become a regular habit and we would not miss having this meal. This highlights the fact that we have been programmed to accept that we all need to have three meals per day, at pre-set times.

Consider the following; if you ordered two meals which were the same (i.e. type and cost), however, when presented to you, one was twice the portion size of the other. Would you automatically choose the bigger portion? If you selected the bigger portion it suggests that your choice has been influenced by your childhood, your 'more is good' habit.

Or, given the choice between having a meal comprising a larger food portion (e.g. a large pasta dish), than one that is smaller (e.g. a fish dish), we will tend to order the bigger portion, especially if it is roughly the same cost. In most cases, this has nothing to do with taste. Our rationale is driven by the fact that we think that the bigger meal will be more 'filling' as we believe that we are hungry. Our food choice has nothing to do with us being hungry as it was our well-established 'more is good' habits influencing our decision.

Our habits and beliefs often mislead us to eat more food than we need. Our 'feel good' moments then make us select unhealthy food choices which aren't ideal for us. When our habits tell us that we are hungry, we will eat almost anything available especially if it is our favourite food.

The good news is that these habits can be changed for good ones. An example of this is that we all know someone who has given up smoking for good. This strongly suggests that if we can give up smoking, we can change our eating habits, and this provides hope for all of us.

Are we really hungry?

I don't believe most people, in modern society, know what the 'real' hungry sensation feels like, as we have been brought up having three meals per day. If we have not eaten for a period (a few hours) and we are feeling weak, this may suggest that we need an intake of food. But this feeling is not real hunger. It is a well-known fact that Mahatma Gandhi survived 21 days without food. [20] If we want to see evidence of hunger, go to rural Africa where the locals may not have had a meal for days at a time.

For most, hunger is an imaginary feeling driven by our habits and beliefs that we need three, regular meals daily. Missing one meal does not mean that we automatically become hungry. This is a complete misconception, a childhood misbelief, and another reason why we overeat.

It is worth considering the following. If our stomach had an automatic warning system with a form of visual indication when it was empty, like our motor car fuel indicator showing us that we are in 'reserve' and we need to fill the tank, then obesity would not be a worldwide issue.

We would be filling our stomach (our tank) only when necessary, which is the underlying theme of the book. If a person, whilst in their childhood, had been told repeatedly that their stomach was an engine, and reference was made to a motor car petrol tank, needing only to be filled up when empty, there is a good chance that they would not be overweight now.

Summary:
- Our childhood influences our future beliefs, habits and behaviour
- Our subconscious mind influences every aspect of our daily life
- Our subconscious process system is based on beliefs, habits and 'feel good' moments
- Most of our daily chores are done completely instinctively, on autopilot
- The subconscious mind plays a significant part in our eating habits
- Our underlying beliefs determine our eating habits
- We are constantly eating in autopilot, without giving our food intake much thought
- Our habits and beliefs often mislead us to eat more food than we need

6. PERSONAL FACTORS THAT INFLUENCE OUR FOOD HABITS (Step 1)

To get a better understanding of how our poor eating habits are created, we need to understand where they came from. There are both personal (i.e. your childhood) and external (i.e. social or environmental) influences that impact our eating habits and harm our good dieting intentions. Personal influences that have shaped our eating habits include:

Unhelpful statements during our childhood

Our parents and teachers, and anyone who was an authority in our early life, had a huge influence on our future eating habits. As children, when it came to food, our minds were trained to accept everything that we were told. Unknown to us, this constant input of instructions had a huge part in all our future habits and beliefs, good or bad.

Whilst in our childhood, we may have heard statements such as:

…. *'you can't leave the table until you finish your plate'*

…. *'you can't have your pudding until you finish your main course'*

…. *'greens are good for you, please eat them up'*

…. *'I am not throwing away good food'*

…. *'wait until your father comes home and I tell him that you have not eaten your greens'*

…. *'there are only two sausages left, I am not throwing them away'*

…. *'we don't waste food, please have the last few potatoes'*

…. *'I am not throwing away good food, I worked hard to put this meal on the table for you'*

Our parents used these statements to help control our food consumption. Fear, guilt and shame are manipulation tools they used to help control our behaviour or get us to do something (e.g. finish your food). Using these statements did not mean that our parents did not love us, they were wanting to make sure we did not go hungry and that the food extras were not wasted.

Most of the above statements had nothing to do with us being hungry, as we had already eaten most of our food portion. Furthermore, there was no need to finish our plate as this may have been our third meal of the day and I am sure our parents would not have let us starve to death.

The underlying message was that, even though we were not hungry, we could carry on eating if we wanted to, a form of validation that 'more is good' and it was an acceptable habit. Eating these extra food portions, having to clear our plate, then became the norm for the rest of our lives.

These statements were constantly programming our minds and shaped our dietary habits. If you are constantly overeating, whether intentional or not, there is a good possibility that the rationale, or cause, goes back to your childhood.

There are examples, that we may not be aware of, which highlight our 'invisible' habits, and these include: We always finish our food on the plate, no matter what. We always volunteer to eat the leftovers in the pot. When in a fast food outlet, we always ask for the biggest burger meal and then 'go-large'. When in a petrol station, we always purchase a treat (sweets) whilst buying fuel. We always have a few biscuits whenever we have a cup of tea.

In most cases, these well-established habits have nothing to do with hunger. We did not need to order the largest burger or finish the leftovers in the pot. We were not born with these 'more is good' eating habits, so they must have come from somewhere. This highlights the fact that we eat like we have always eaten. These are established eating habits that we need to change if we don't want to experience another dieting failure.

It is worth noting that if our parents were to have put the words 'don't have to' in front of most of the above statements, there would be a good chance that we would not now be reading this book.

Other unhelpful statements

Other statements that we may have heard from our parents when we were a kid include:

…. *'he has always liked his food'*

…. *'she has always had a sweet tooth'*

…. *'when it comes to eating, she takes after her father'*

…. *'he is always hungry'*

Most would confirm that there is no logical truth in these statements. These statements, and beliefs, were passed down to us by our parents to ensure that we did not feel guilty when challenged about our excessive food consumption (e.g. eating sweets) and providing a form of justification for the position we find ourselves in at the time (i.e. being overweight). We simply accepted these statements and have had to live with them for most of our lives, providing a convenient excuse for another dieting failure.

If we still believe that there is an element of truth in these statements, these beliefs, then we are misinformed. Accept that they are incorrect, as they could still be influencing our food habits and the possible reasons for our dieting failures.

An interesting observation of a statement that did not work. When our parents told us that eating sweets will 'rot our teeth and make them fall out', we did not believe them. Perhaps this was because sweets may have been previously given to us as a reward, on a regular basis, a reassurance that they were okay to eat.

Perfect mummy/daddy syndrome.

When parents were keen to show you how much they loved you, and how perfect their parenting skills were, they tended to have an approach of 'more food is good for you'. It is common to see the food portion on the child's plate is the same, or even greater than their parents, even though the child is considerably smaller in physical size and shape.

Those early portion sizes determined what we consider is normal. If our mother served us a pasta dish that took us 40 to 50 mouthfuls to finish, this habit will now be accepted as the norm and this will set a precedent for the rest of our lives. As a kid, how would we know if 30 or even 20 mouthfuls would have been more than adequate?

Our parents may have also said the following:

.... 'you must be really hungry as you have been out playing football all afternoon, so I will add more food to your plate'.

I don't believe that there is any logical truth to this as we should only be eating when we are hungry, not when our mother thinks that we should be. If our mother has always only served us 30 mouthfuls of pasta, there is no reason why we should have extra just because we spent the afternoon running around a field chasing a football. We don't 'top-up' the fuel tank of our motor car when we have been for a longer than usual drive.

These unhelpful beliefs, introduced by others, provide us with another excuse to overeat.

Temptation (forbidden treats)

When we walk past a bakery, or restaurant, and smell or see an eye-pleasing display, this can be a huge temptation for us. [21] Is this because, when we were kids, our parents highlighted this fact with the following statements?

.... 'look at that beautiful cake on display, it must taste very nice'

.... 'smell that bread, it must taste yummy'

In most cases, a visit to the cake shop was a reward for good behaviour, given to us by our 'perfect' parents, and usually associated with an occasion, or a day out. This habit that we have inherited, can be difficult to ignore and isn't just triggered by taste or smell, there is a nostalgic 'feel good' moment. As a child, this nostalgia overcame any logical explanation as to why we should not eat this food treat.

This desire to indulge in these food temptations, when we were children, extends into adulthood, providing another reason for us to fail on our latest diet.

'What the hell, let's just do it' moments

When we were a child, we may have heard the following statement from our parents:

.... *'what the hell, let's just do it'*.

This is a strong emotion inherited from our childhood which influences our behavioural habits and plays a significant role in our attitude to eating. This statement is used when we want to overcome a feeling of guilt or we are in a helpless situation. We are wanting some form of justification for our actions, so we experience one of those 'what the hell, let's just do it' moments, as we don't want to accept responsibility for our actions.

We try to overcome these episodes with a 'feel good' moment and we generally head for the fridge for a quick snack or go out for a treat in a restaurant, or bar, leading to us overeat and consume more alcohol than we should. This perceived dieting failure is likely to trigger further negative emotions which will cause us to overindulge on our favourite foods.

Holiday and alcoholic 'feel good' binges

Whilst on holiday or socialising with friends, when we are in a relaxed mode, we experience 'feel good' moments. We switch off any logic, or rational, reasoning that we may have, and we tend to binge on excessive food and drink. We constantly experience our 'what the hell, let's just do it' moments.

A good example of this is when we are in hotels offering all-inclusive meal offers. At mealtimes, when we are at home, we typically only have one plateful of food. However, we now think it is acceptable to have three platefuls of food at one sitting, before having a dessert.

Typically, the more alcohol we drink, the more we eat. Even though we have eaten a lovely meal, by the time we get home we may consider a snack before bed. In the morning, feeling slightly hung-over, we then indulge in a full breakfast and top-up, with a few slices of toast and jam, even though most mornings we would not consider having a large breakfast.

These habits have been inherited from our parents, or later in life from our peer groups. Having seen them enjoy themselves, by overindulging on food and alcohol, there is a good chance that we will do the same. These sequences of events are linked. To enjoy ourselves, we need to overeat and drink more than usual.

These 'feel good' binges are a nightmare for anyone on a weight loss programme. If we are serious about wanting to lose weight, we must reduce or eliminate these 'what the hell, let's just do it' moments.

Distraction whilst eating

When distracted whilst eating, such as when we are talking, watching TV, texting, or playing video games, this could lead us to overeat, as we are not aware of the amount of food entering our bodies.

For some families, it is rare that they all sit down at the dining table to eat their meal. Mealtimes now consist of kids taking their food to their room to eat, whilst watching TV or playing video games. We often see families, sitting in a restaurant, who are all totally addicted to their mobile telephones whilst eating.

If we are so preoccupied doing other things, whilst we are eating, then why are we eating such large meals? It is obvious that we are not experiencing the pleasure or the taste of our food. We are eating the whole plate full of food because it is there and who cares how many calories we have just eaten? Meals have now become a non-important event and we are creating unhealthy eating habits for our children.

Have we been conned?

Most parents, going back 40 to 50 years, were not familiar with food portion control, what foods were good or bad for you, or familiar with diets. In most cases, the overall range of healthy foods was limited, and the daily food intake was very basic, dictated by what was affordable at the time.

All the above suggests we may have all been conned, as most of our beliefs to justify our eating habits, are not factual or were not backed-up by science. We are all products of our parent's lack of food-awareness. Unfortunately, most of us are now passing on our beliefs and habits to our children. This has been confirmed by the continual increase in worldwide obesity rates.

Habits in adulthood

Not all our eating habits have been adopted from our childhood, passed on from our parents. Habits can be created in an instant, especially if there is logical justification (e.g. it is free) and there is a reward (i.e. a treat).

For example, coffee shops, such as Costa and Starbucks, are a regular feature in our lives and visits to these outlets are now a daily habit. If one of these outlets opened nearby, this will result in you consuming more coffee and cakes, than before. As it is now convenient for you to visit these coffee shops and you consider it a treat.

If you work in the public care industry, such as veterinary surgeries, or care homes, there will be a constant supply of free boxes of biscuits and chocolates left behind by clients. Previously, you may have not considered yourself to have an excessive chocolate habit, however, as these are now free, you will indulge, whenever there is an opportunity.

Eating 'on the move'

Our busy, hectic, stressful lives mean we are regularly eating 'on the move'. When we are in this eating mode, we are not concentrating, or appreciating, what we are eating. During these times, we have a complete detachment from our thought process and what we are putting into our mouths. In some cases, we can't remember what we had to eat. In these instances, are we hungry, or are we just eating the food as we have a train to catch to go to our next meeting?

In these scenarios, we have a complete disconnect with our 'real' hunger. We are not listening to our bodies, resulting in us eating more than we should.

Boredom and the influence on eating habits

Another habit adopted in adulthood is eating out of boredom, or pointless eating. Boredom is a common emotional state that most people experience from time to time. Without meaningful stimulus and focus, we experience emptiness, worthlessness, loneliness or have a lack of interest in the activity that we are engaged in. This lack of stimulation leaves us craving relief which could lead us to indulge in activities that could have behavioural and social consequences.

It has been well researched that boredom plays a large role in creating addictions such as drugs, alcohol, gambling and watching pornography. Some may say that it is 'the root of all sin'. If we were constantly busy and living a meaningful life, there should be no time to indulge in these pastimes.

One of the options, to break the boredom, is to consume food or drink that we don't need. In most cases people eat, or drink alcohol, to break the monotony, rather than for the pleasure. These 'fixes' will create long-term habits/addictions which may be difficult to break.

For some, identifying when we are eating out of boredom, may be difficult. However, in most cases, this should be easy to identify as typically this occurs when having 'in-between' meals, outside our regular meals.

Our adopted eating habits, in adulthood, have nothing to do with our upbringing, as these opportunities were not around when we were a child. They have now become norms that lead to us eating more than we should, resulting in an increase in calories entering our bodies daily.

Summary:
- The subconscious mind plays a significant part in our eating habits
- Our eating habits were created in our childhood and shaped by emotions such as fear, guilt and shame
- Our food intake habits are influenced by 'feel good' moments
- The 'what the hell, let's just do it' moments are habits that help us justify our food intake
- For most of our childhood, we had a limited say in the food portions

that were served to us

- When distracted, or eating-on the move, this could lead to excessive food consumption
- Food habits and beliefs can be created in an instant
- Boredom could be a cause for overeating

7. EXTERNAL (SOCIAL) FACTORS WHICH INFLUENCE OUR FOOD HABITS (Step 1)

There are several external social factors that influence our food intake habits, most of which are unintentional and not within our control. Without realising, we are now all eating much more than we used to and there are several reasons for this.

Supermarket influences on our food intake

Supermarkets play a significant role in our daily lives and most of us visit these places on a regular basis. They are under constant pressure to make the food they sell (e.g. ready meals) healthy and nutritious. They have been previously criticized for the high carbohydrate, salt, fat, sugar content in their foods, however, this has improved.

We are generally attracted to foods that have eye-catching packaging or recently advertised. If the same food item was displayed without packaging, would we be still attracted? We may also purchase the item if it's endorsed by a celebrity on TV. This often leads us to purchase the item, even though, when we walked into the supermarket, we had no intention of buying the product.

Examples of this are 'bog offs', the buy one and get one free sale offers; or the 'fine meal deals', a three-course meal with a bottle of wine at a perceived cheap price. For most, these offers may sound like a bargain. However, we are potentially increasing our consumption by 30 to 40%, adding additional mouthfuls, on food that we were not planning to have in the first place. Recent research shows that around 70% of shoppers, who took advantage of these 'bog offs', are obese, which suggests that, for the supermarkets, their sales strategies are working. [22]

The 'ready meals' that supermarkets sell have grown in size over the years. Research by the British Heart Foundation shows that a beef lasagne ready meal has increased by 39%, a curry meal by 50% and a chicken pie by 40%. [23] If the supermarkets were to sell smaller portions, we would reduce obesity overnight. In my opinion, aeroplane food is smaller in portion size when compared to an average 'ready meal', yet we don't hear passengers complaining when they are presented with their meal.

Furthermore, supermarkets over-size their products. Why do we have to purchase six sausages when we only want four? As a result, we cook all six sausages as we don't want to waste the food. This leads to families, our kids, having to eat these extra sausages leading to overeating and creating habits or norms that will be around for the rest of their lives.

Another example is the selling of multi-pack options, such as chocolate bars (e.g. Mars bars). Instead of buying our child one portion, like in the old days, we are now buying packs containing twelve bars. The result is that there is now large supply of chocolate bars in our kitchen, for our children to eat whenever they want, creating another habit for life. Given the choice, they will opt for a chocolate bar rather than a portion of fruit that is healthier.

Supermarkets have been determining our portion sizes for most of our lives. They believed that 'more is good', as this means, at a small additional unit cost to us, they will improve their turnover. Their annual reporting of their financial turnover, to their shareholders, is their main motivation, not our health or wellbeing.

Restaurant food portions

In most restaurants, they believe that 'more on the plate' is good for business. In most cases, we don't have a say in the food portion sizes they serve us, even though we are paying for the meal. We will always finish the plateful, even if it's a bigger food portion than normal. If we don't finish the plate of food, we consider it a misuse of our hard-earned money. Overeating, in this instance, means we are treating our body as a waste disposal bin, another method of dumping the excess food that we don't need to eat.

When at home most of us don't have a starter, or a dessert, after our main meal. However, when we enter a restaurant and the menu is placed in front of us, we are programmed to order a starter, have our main meal and then a dessert. The result is that we are increasing the volume of food entering our bodies by around 40 to 50%. If we don't have a starter and a dessert at home, why do we have to order these when in a restaurant?

It is estimated that a third (33%) of all Americans eat out every day and the average adult dines out at a restaurant five to six times a week. [24] As we have limited control of our food consumption, when visiting a restaurant, this suggests that it is one of the main reasons why the average American calorie intake is greater than in most countries.

Takeaway foods

Takeaways meals are now a regular feature in our lives, providing us with a large selection of food that can be enjoyed in the comfort of our home. The main attraction is that they are convenient, tasty, perceived to be cheap and there is no food preparation required.

Typically, we associate takeaway food with high-fat, carbohydrate type foods, such as pizza, curry, chips, etc. However, over the years, the sector has responded to criticism and there is now a demand for healthier foods, such as low-fat, low-carb food, especially in larger cities.

The total foodservice delivery market was worth around £8.5 billion in 2019 [25] and there has been a 34% increase in growth from 2010 to 2018. [26] With the emergence of online ordering, the sector is forecast to grow even further.

Research suggests that people who are more exposed to nearby takeaway outlets are nearly twice as likely to be obese. [27] In some instances, our children are having a takeaway meal daily. It is a worrying trend, especially for those who are already obese.

The main issue is that these meal portions are generally larger in size and have greater calorie content when compared to a similar-sized meal, prepared at home. Furthermore, they don't come with any calorie content information on the packaging. For anyone who is regularly eating having takeaways, it will be a challenge to not overeat and exceed your daily recommended calorie allowance.

Fast food portions sizes

Fast food outlets are now big business and globally the industry generates revenue of over $570 (£450) billion annually. The growth rate of fast food outlets in the USA alone has increased from $6 (£4.8) billion in 1970 to $200 (£160) billion in 2015? [28]

The size of an average burger has significantly increased over the years. In 1955 the average burger was 104 grams (3.7 oz), now it is 260 grams (9.2 oz). [29] This represents an increase of 150% of the original size. When we enter a fast food outlet, we are now presented with an option of not just one, but two or even three burger patties in the same bun. Not only are the burgers now much bigger, the add-on toppings such as bacon, cheese, salad and sauces are well-established options. This all leads to an increase in the overall calories.

The portion size of French fries has increased since 1955, from 68 grams (2.4 oz) to 167 grams (5.9 oz), a 145% increase. Their sugary drinks (e.g. Coke) were 207ml (7 fl oz) and are now 887ml (30 fl oz), a 328% increase. [30]

It is now standard practice to ask us if we want to turn our order into a meal, to include French fries and a sugary drink, or to 'go large', to increase the size of the portion of chips and sugary drink. When accepting their 'amazing meal' offer, this all leads to a significant increase in the overall calories for our meal.

These promotions are targeting our kids and members of society who may not be well-educated and find it hard to say no. This is an important part of their sales strategy. Their plan is to 're-educate' or re-programme our minds so that large portion sizes are acceptable, and it is now the normal size for an adult or teenager. This belief will extend through their teenage years and into adulthood.

Most would confirm that eating a burger (500 to 600 kcal) on its own is acceptable, as they contain protein and some salad. It is the add-ons that increase our overall calorie intake to unacceptable levels, especially for children.

If the portions we were eating 30 years ago were enough, why are we now eating 100 to 150% more calories per meal? Human beings, during this time, have not grown or altered in genetic make-up or physical structure. This is not our choice and we have never been consulted on these increases in food and drink portion sizes that have been forced upon us.

It is obvious that the objective of fast food corporations is, if they cannot persuade us to eat two burgers a day, the next alternative is to increase the unit portion size. They want us to eat more, as an extra 50 pence/cents on the average burger meal is a significant revenue generator and will increase their annual financial turnover.

They are certainly not thinking about our wellbeing, the worldwide obesity issues, or the long-term associated health costs that we may have when we get older.

Fig 1: How our burger sizes have evolved

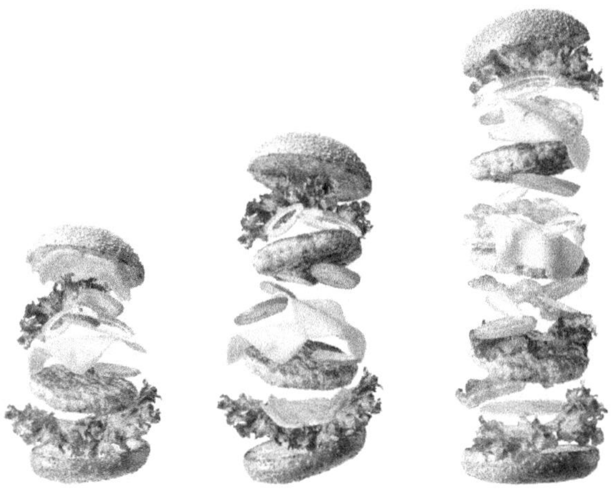

Media advertising influencing our long-term food habits

Media and television play a significant part in shaping our subconscious mind. Food advertising is designed to reassure us that their product is nutritious, good financial value and provides a validation mechanism to get their positive message over to the public. They know that constant, repeated advertising will eventually change our food habits, resulting in an increase in revenue for them.

Research has shown that exposure to unhealthy foods through constant TV marketing has been linked to increased preferences for marketed foods, especially in children. [31] For most people, if it has been on TV, it must be okay. They can't dissociate the fact that it is another advertisement promoting a company's products.

For the average American, the media (TV advertising) has a massive influence on reassuring them that large food portions are the norm. It is common to see TV advertisements for 16-inch sized pizzas targeting teenagers. Most teenagers in the rest of the world have never seen a 16-inch pizza.

Television cooking shows

Most of us now spend hours watching TV cooking shows, presented by gurus with 'god-like' status. Most of the meals that they prepare are generous in portion size as they can't be seen to be offering small food portions on TV.

Media and visual presentation play a significant part in shaping our subconscious mind, reinforcing our beliefs that, having seen it on TV, everyone else must be eating the same larger-sized meals.

Summary:
- Meal portions provided by third parties (e.g. supermarkets, fast food outlets and restaurants) have increased in size without us having noticed
- Third parties play a huge part in portion size and our daily food intake
- Media advertising influence our food habits
- Most of us have now accepted these large-sized portions as the norm
- These external factors, over which we have limited control, result in us eating more food than we should

8. REHAB OUR EATING HABITS (Step 2)

Step two of The Rehab Weight Loss Plan:

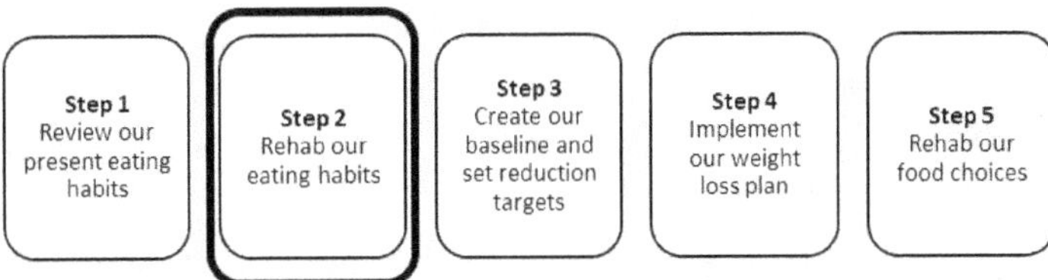

We are now aware that our well-established eating habits are sabotaging our good dieting intentions and they originate from various personal and social factors. To ensure that we don't 'default' back into our usual dieting cycle, we need to re-think our eating habits. We need to have a different rationale for our food consumption, to make sure that we are not eating in autopilot or letting third parties dictate our food choices.

Our 'more is good' eating habits are causing us to overeat on a regular basis. To change the status quo, we need to rehab our eating habits, re-programme our subconscious mind. Our objective is to introduce new 'less is good' habits to make sure our old ones don't re-surface.

Acceptance that our subconscious mind is influencing our eating habits

An important part of the habit-changing process is identifying the fact that our current habits are an issue and we need a good reason for changing these. We now know that these 'invisible' habits are dictating our food intake and we need to accept that they are real and need to be changed.

Not all the underlying causes, personal and social, may directly apply to you, but most would indirectly have an influence on your food intake, such as from third parties. If you don't accept these facts, you can't move-on to the next stage.

Our main motivation for changing our ways, our reward, is that we will achieve our long-term weight loss and wellbeing goals, which is our main objective.

What do we need to break our old habits?

Now that we recognize the role that the subconscious mind plays when shaping our eating habits, it is possible to re-programme (rehab) our thought processes, through simple mind-changing exercises. Changing our eating habits isn't easy, but once a habit has been changed it becomes a way of life.

When starting a new diet, we are trying to force new habits on top of old, well-established ones introduced to us by our parents, those in authority and third-party influences (e.g. media). If these new habits are seen to be too radical (e.g. a low-carb diet that may make us feel nauseous), or restrictive (e.g. we can't eat our favourite foods), then these will be resisted, causing another dieting failure. Also, it needs to be a small habit change, not a major one (e.g. eating food that is not familiar to you).

In most cases, if we believe that we do not have to greatly sacrifice or deviate from our daily habits, this will make it easier to change. On the Rehab Weight Loss plan, we are not asking you to give up your favourite foods as this is part of the habit-changing process. Furthermore, it is a 'small' habit-change, as our objective is to reduce our mouthfuls, have smaller portions and this should not prove to be a major change in your eating habits.

Most of us, over time, have changed certain eating habits when we felt they were not good for us or were a risk to our wellbeing. There are numerous examples of these changes; we stopped using butter and started cooking with virgin olive oil, we stopped putting teaspoons of sugar in our tea, we changed our bread-type for healthy multi-grain options. These changes were all driven by our desire to eat healthier and the belief that we would lose weight. These habit changes would have taken place over a short period, say, in one to three days.

Most people know someone who has given up a lifelong smoking habit. Smoking is a classic example of a habit that was adopted along the way.

If our parents smoked, there is a good chance that we may start smoking. As our parents enjoyed smoking, they would not have highlighted the long-term dangers and we would have accepted that it is okay to smoke. Further validation was confirmed by advertisements, via TV or billboards, highlighting a 'feel good' moment if we smoked. We all now know the dangers of smoking, so most of us don't smoke.

If we can give up a highly addictive habit, such as smoking, this suggests that our eating habits can be changed if we have willpower and apply the habit changing strategies in this book.

Most would agree that reducing our mouthfuls at each meal will be much easier than having to stop smoking. If you are having reservations about whether you will be able to change our old eating habits, then let this be a motivating statement.

Time-period to change a habit

The period to change a habit will vary depending on your motivation, the rationale and degree of complexity. Most importantly, does the person operate in a subconscious mode for most of their life, constantly procrastinating and not getting things done? In this scenario, it will take time to implement a new habit.

Someone who is constantly aware of their actions, is in a conscious mode for most of the time and is interested in improving their wellbeing, will have a better chance of introducing a new healthy habit, in a shorter period. Also, to change a habit, we need to repeat the underlying message as often as possible. For example, if the habit we are wanting to change only takes place once per week, then this will be a challenge to break.

When changing an eating habit, we would, on most days, be having five to seven different meals (including snacks). This means that we now have five to seven chances, every day, to constantly challenge the rationale for eating these large meals, so we should see a rapid change in our habits, especially if the reward is long-term weight loss.

The overall sacrifice (i.e. to eat less of our favourite meals) is small compared to the reward (i.e. achieving our goal weight and improved wellbeing). To succeed, to change our eating habits, we only need the desire to lose weight and the self-discipline to stay on the plan.

Remove negative emotions that sabotage our good intentions

To start the process, we need to be looking at the bigger picture and have a more realistic view of ourselves, so we can see the positives in our lives. If we are constantly filling our lives with negative feelings about our self-worth, our body weight, then we need to change this. For example, if you have a well-established belief that you will always be 'fat', and there is nothing you can do about it, there is a good chance no diet will help you.

There is no such thing as someone being lazy, greedy, needy, or unmotivated. To use hurtful words such as these requires some form of comparison against other third parties and are difficult to quantify. Someone has told us this when we were a kid and we have just accepted it. These phrases were used to manipulate us, to get us to alter our behaviour or do something that they wanted.

Furthermore, we must accept that we are not always perfect. Being perfect is wanting to compare ourselves with others. Accept that everyone is different and that being perfect is an imaginary, non-achievable thought in our minds.

We can always find excuses to overeat or drink too much. These are excuses and if we are going to move forward, we need to acknowledge that this is what they are. When we are constantly damaging our attempts to lose weight with excuses, we are undermining our hopes of removing the depression and helplessness that we feel when overweight.

We must improve our self-image to one that reflects who we are or want to be. In most cases, our negative thoughts are linked to our past and have created insecurities that may live with us forever. Losing weight makes us feel healthier, gives us a positive outlook and we become more confident. Why would we want to sabotage these positive feelings by a negative comment from someone else in our youth?

To start the process, we need to 'clear the slate', clear our mind of negative beliefs or habits that may interfere with the process. We are going to let new ideas and, more importantly, new healthy habits enter our lives. We need to accept that we alone are responsible for what goes into our mouth. We alone can decide if we want to change our eating habits.

Fig 2: Yes, you can do it

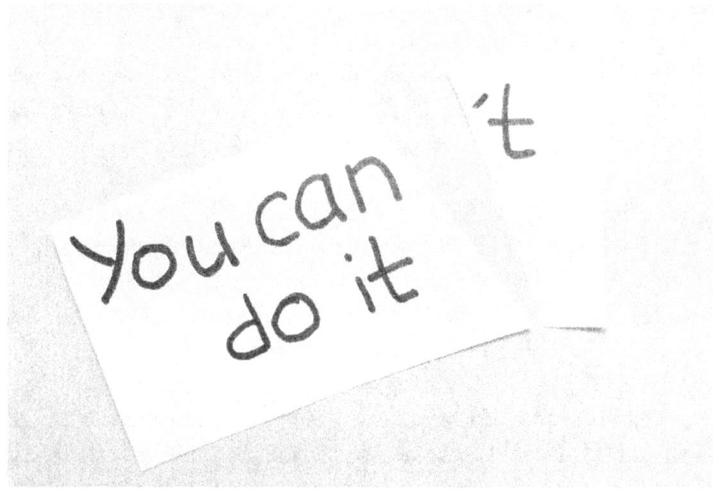

Identifying the reasons for overeating

We all need to eat on a regular basis to maintain our energy levels to get us through the day. When we are having larger than normal meals, resulting in us overeating, we need to identify what the underlying factors are, what is causing us to do this.

In most cases, as we are constantly eating in autopilot, we have never considered why we are eating the meal. Understanding what our rationale is for eating larger than normal-sized meals will help us recognise what we must do to change the process. This is an important part of the rehab of our subconscious thought process.

The possible reasons for eating larger portions of food than normal are:

- It is our favourite meal and it has become a habit that we adopted
- It is a misbelief that certain foods are good for us
- It was a social event leading to excessive food and alcohol consumption
- An offer from a third party and it was free

41

- We were feeling depressed due to external factors or family issues
- It was a treat which we deserved as we recently had a hard time
- It was a 'what the hell, let's just do it' or a 'feel good' moment
- We have never put any thought into why we had that meal

Most of the above reasons are established habits that we have adopted. Accepting our habit(s), by not denying them, will make us more aware of our rationale when it comes to overeating.

Having identified why, when and where these dieting failures are taking place, the easiest option is to avoid the scenario completely. However, as the objective of the Rehab Weight Loss Plan is to change our eating habits, there should be no reason why we can't still do what we normally enjoy, like eating our favourite meal or attending a social event.

If our new diet is seen as too much of a sacrifice, then there is a possibility that it will fail. However, if we are serious about wanting to lose weight, we will require some willpower and we are going to have to decide what is more important, our long-term wellbeing or the potential distraction (e.g. social events) that may harm our good intentions.

Excessive eating and drinking amongst the younger generation have more to do with ego and emotional intelligence, a complete disconnect of the mind and body. Not eating a portion of food on our plate, or ordering a dessert, or having another bottle of wine, should not be considered a 'big deal' to us or our friends. We were there for the social occasion and not for an eating or drinking competition as to who can consume the most.

Where we have been experiencing personal issues (e.g. home or work-related stress), then we need to identify that these are not justifiable reasons to eat more than usual or choose unhealthy options. It's another one of those habits that we have adopted to conveniently justify the rationale for eating a takeaway or similar meal.

We need to accept that these negative influences could have long-term mental consequences. These issues should not be linked to our eating habits as they are not justifiable reasons. Overeating, in these instances, will only worsen our emotional circumstances.

Simple avoidance statements

We have now identified why, when and where our eating habits are taking place and causing our dieting failures. However, if we are still constantly making excuses (the 'what the hell, let's just do it' moments), then consider using the following statement when presented with a potential cause for another dieting failure.

… 'No social event or negative emotion should ever influence my food intake'.

There is a good chance that we have never linked our circumstances (e.g. social events or personal issues) to our overeating. Now we know there is a connection, we need to repeat the above statement on a regular basis, as this will help us in overcoming these distractions.

Why do we eat?

The primary reason we eat is to have enough energy for our bodies to function and that we are not hungry. This is driven by our beliefs and habits that we need to eat at least three meals daily.

There are other secondary 'triggers' (e.g. personal and social factors); such as a smell or taste temptation, a 'feel good' moment', supermarket sales offer, a freebie, or alcohol-induced, to name a few, which also influence our rationale for wanting to eat. The justification for these 'triggers' is our established beliefs and our 'more is good' habits that we have adopted.

Once we start eating, we move into autopilot mode. This means that we have limited control of the volume of food entering our bodies, as we have eaten the same meals hundreds of times.

It is worth noting that some 815 million people in the world, around one in nine, do not have enough food to lead a healthy active life. [32] These secondary 'triggers', mean nothing to these unfortunate people, as most of these opportunities are not available to them. This suggests that these 'triggers' are only a luxury for most of us in the developed world.

This point highlights the fact that we are not born with these secondary 'triggers', we don't need them to survive, and we will not go hungry without them. This strongly suggests that we can change our beliefs, our 'more is good' eating habits so that they don't influence our food intake daily.

To change our existing habits, so that these secondary 'triggers' have limited influence, we need to disconnect our mind, our rationale for food, from our stomachs. Unless there is a disconnection, we will constantly be eating more than what our bodies need.

My body is an engine

We have always associated our hunger, our rationale for eating, with our stomach. To change this thought process, we need to constantly refer our stomach as an engine, a mechanical 'thing' with no emotions, habits, or beliefs.

We always relate the operation of our car engine with the petrol tank and we only fill-up with fuel when it is empty. We need to treat our food intake the same. We only put food (fuel) into our stomach (petrol tank) when it is a necessity.

Our food calories are the same as a litre of fuel, a unit of energy. To save fuel (energy) we need to reduce the amount entering our engine. When there is less going into our bodies, this means that there is less food for our stomachs to process, or store as body fat.

The performance of our engine should never be influenced by our beliefs, our secondary 'triggers', food temptations, or the latest supermarket offers.

This simple change in our thought process is an important part of the overall habit-changing process.

Fig 3: My body is an engine

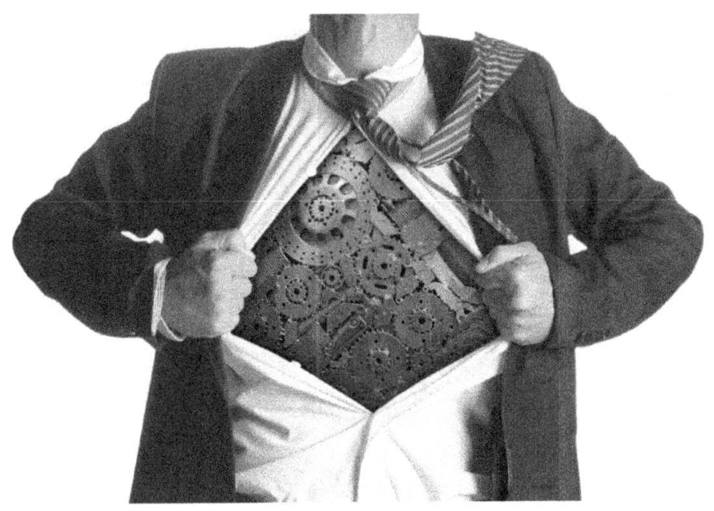

Verbal repetition of a positive message to change habits

Knowing the reasons why, when and where we are overeating, we need to constantly challenge these habits and find methods of 'breaking' out of our autopilot mode when eating. Research has shown that using verbal repetition of a positive message can help re-programme our subconscious mind and change our habits to healthy ones. [33]

We have all done this before at various stages of our lives. An example of this is when we were studying for an exam at school. We would go over and over the same relevant fact until it was 'fixed' in our brain, our memory, for good. Like entering information into a computer waiting to be used sometime in the future.

When there was a potentially life-threatening issue (i.e. an electrical shock, or crossing the road), our parents would have constantly repeated this message that we need to be careful when operating electrical equipment or crossing the road. As we are all now aware of these potential dangers, this suggests that this habit changing method does work as they are all now well-established habits.

We need to disrupt our thought process by disconnecting our food intake from our established 'more is good' habits. This is the reason why we need to treat our stomach like an engine, a 'mechanical thing'. I am refuelling my engine and not my well-established habit.

We need to regularly challenge our food intake, to prevent us from eating out of habit, by using the following statements:

.... *'my body is an engine. Am I feeding another habit of mine or am I really hungry?'*

.... *'does my engine really need to have this large meal?'*

.... *'is my engine still enjoying this meal?'*

.... *'why am I eating more than my engine needs?'*

.... *'does my engine really need to finish my plate of food?*

.... *'why are they serving my engine all this food, there must be 60 to 80 mouthfuls on this plate?'*

...... *'my engine has already had 100 mouthfuls today, why do I need more?'*

By constantly challenging our subconscious thought process, when presented with a large meal, we will quickly see a change in our habits. This simple change in our thought process, referring to our stomach as an engine, will help change our rationale for wanting to finish large food portions.

When do we stop tasting our food?

Knowing when to stop eating is the biggest challenge for anyone on a diet. If we could simply push the 'off' button at any time this would help us reduce our food intake. However, as we are in the subconscious mode most of the time, whilst we are eating, we are not aware of the number of mouthfuls entering our body. Furthermore, as we have never been told how much is enough, this makes it even harder for us to just switch off.

To help us stop eating, by reducing the mouthfuls entering our bodies (our engine), we need to send a positive, supportive, motivating message to our minds to help us stop.

In my opinion, we do not taste our food after three to five mouthfuls of most meals. I am not aware of any specific scientific research to back up this fact. My guess is that, after the first few mouthfuls, our mind goes back into subconscious or autopilot mode. There is some logic to this as we have been eating food every day and our mind has been operating in autopilot mode for most of this time.

To confirm this, it is suggested that you carry out this experiment for yourselves. This will provide the reassurance and the rationale that you need to help justify your change of habit, to stop you from overeating.

A simple way of helping us stop overeating, when we are presented with a large meal, is to remind ourselves of the following message:

.... *'if I cannot taste my food after five mouthfuls, why am I still eating this meal?'*

Let this positive statement be our main motivating, supporting message to help stop us from overeating when presented with a large food portion.

The Rehab 'less is good' habit change strategy

To simplify the above, to make our habit-changing process easier, consider using the following statements, when presented with a large meal:

.... *'why am I eating this large meal? Is it another habit of mine?'*

.... *'if I can't taste my food after five mouthfuls, why am I still eating this meal?'*

..... *'having a larger food portion does not mean I am enjoying my food more'*

Consider repeating these simple statements every time we are presented with a large meal and, with time, we will start seeing a new, good eating habit established. With these statements, we are first challenging the importance of having the meal, and then providing a justifiable reason for not eating the whole portion.

If we carry out this simple, habit-changing strategy several times daily, and we are constantly reducing the size of our food portions, we will be creating a new 'less is good' habit. The reward is that we will soon experience weight loss.

As our eating habits influence every aspect of our daily food consumption, we need to appreciate why we need to change our thought process. Our future success on the Rehab Weight Loss Plan, or any other diet, will depend on how we disconnect our eating habits from our food intake (our fuel) that we are about to put in our bodies (our engine).

It is worth noting that if our parents had encouraged us to use these supporting statements when we were children, there would be a good chance that we would not be reading this book.

Self-congratulation

In our childhood, an important part of the habit-forming process was the reward, the constant positive reassurance from our parents that our behaviour was acceptable. It is important that we congratulate ourselves when we have done something positive (e.g. we are constantly challenging our eating habits) or we achieved a milestone (i.e. weight loss).

As we are now an adult, there is a good chance that no-one else will reward our dieting achievements. With regular self-congratulation, our new habit will become second nature.

For example, having achieved our daily mouthful reduction targets, consider congratulating ourselves with statements like:

…. *'this diet is easy, I can do this, well-done'*

…. *'I am eating smaller meals now, this is not a major sacrifice, I can do this'*

If we enjoy treats (e.g. a chocolate bar), then consider giving ourselves a treat at the end of the week, once we have achieved a weight loss milestone. However, be careful, we could be creating another bad habit.

How do we know we will not go back to our old habits?

Research shows that through some simple mind exercises we can re-programme our minds to disrupt our mind-set or thinking process. [34] On the first stage of the Rehab Weight Loss Plan, we can still eat our normal, favourite meals, so this sacrifice is not exactly a life-changing decision. Also, the new habit changes are small ones, not major changes to our eating habits (e.g. food we don't like). So, we should not be using this as an excuse, and we need to constantly reassure ourselves of this fact.

Previously, when we failed whilst on a diet, we blamed the dieting method, intentionally or not. It is always easier to blame a third-party or the process than to accept our own failures. As we are establishing a new rationale for eating food, having removed our old ones, we have no-one else to blame but ourselves.

If we believe that we can't live without larger-sized food portions, then our food intake is still dictated by our beliefs, and our 'more is good' habits.

The fact that we are now thinking about this, and constantly challenging the rationale for our food intake, is a good start. We will soon see a shift in mindset and, for the first time in our lives, we will be in control of our daily food intake. The positive changes are a very strong emotion and will help drive us forward and keep us on our weight loss plan.

My experience:

It took me around a week before noticing the difference in my rationale for food and I now believe that I have totally changed my eating habits. My new 'less is good' habits don't dictate my hunger. I am not eating in autopilot mode and these new habits will be with me for life.

I have noticed that my food awareness has improved, and I am not eating for the sake of it. I am constantly looking at the bigger picture and reminding myself that the meal I am about to have is greater than 5 to 10 mouthfuls. I have found that a starter-sized meal is just as nice as a larger portioned meal. I don't need a large meal to satisfy my perceived hunger.

Occasionally, when I do veer-off the rails and have a 'blow out', a larger than a normal meal, the difference now is that I have the tools to self-correct, as I am more aware of my habits.

Summary:
- To help break old habits, we need to be aware of what caused them
- We need to re-programme (rehab) our eating habits
- No social event or negative emotion should ever influence our food intake
- We need to treat our body as an engine
- When changing a habit, a verbal repetition of a positive message is an important part of the process
- To help us change our 'more is good' habits, we need to constantly challenge the necessity of having larger-sized meal
- When presented with a larger than normal-sized food portion, always use the Rehab habit-changing strategy to challenge the justification of the large meal

9. ALTERNATIVE HABIT CHANGING METHOD (Step 2)

A simple search on the internet will highlight several different habit changing methods. One well-established method of changing a habit is meditation.

To be successful, on the Rehab Weight Loss Plan, we don't necessarily have to practice meditation. However, for some who may be finding it a challenge to break their 'more is good' habits, then simple meditation exercises may help.

Using meditation to drive home the message

Meditation is a method of transforming our mind so that a new positive message can help change our habits and beliefs. [35]

When practicing any form of meditation, our objective is to focus our mind on the present, paying attention to what we are doing now. This frees the mind from distraction, stress, anxiety and depression. By concentrating on the 'now', all our negative thoughts are set aside, and we have the time to surround ourselves with positive thoughts.

Typically, we need a quiet relaxing room and around 10 to 15 minutes of 'me' time, with no distraction from the telephone, kids, dogs, or partner. A good time of day is either first thing in the morning, before getting out of bed, or the last thing at night.

To carry out the meditation process we need to:

- Lie down on a bed completely still and close our eyes
- Make sure that our concentration is not interrupted or distracted
- Focus on our breathing, so we can hear and feel the motion of our chest
- Starting at our toes, concentrate on the area and start relaxing it (to feel weightlessness)
- Move up through our body, repeating the same exercise
- Once our whole body feels 'free' from outside distractions and is relaxed, then we can start applying simple positive messages

Our message must be a positive one and focused on 'me' and my future goals.

- My body is an engine
- I need to constantly monitor my consumption
- I am not going to let my old habits dictate my food intake
- As I can still eat all my favourite meals, my reduction of mouthfuls is not a great sacrifice. I can do this
- I am the only person who can control my food consumption intake
- I will not be obsessed with other people's opinions
- 'More is not good', 'Less is good'
- With my reduction in food intake, I will lose weight and I am going to feel great
- No people, events or third parties (such as fast food outlets), are going to influence my eating habits
- Future visualisation. Consider how you will look with your 'new' body and how your overall wellbeing will improve

For people who have never carried out any form of meditation, it will take time to get in 'tune' with your body. If you are having a problem 'connecting', then repeat the procedure many times until you feel yourself relaxing and you are in full control of your mind.

We are not suggesting that we spend the rest of our life practising meditation, however, in the first week or two, there may be a need to reconfirm the positive message again and again so that we don't give up our weight loss plan.

How do we know when the message is starting to work?

People who practise various forms of meditation soon see the positive benefits and are happier, more content with life and are healthier in body and mind. Re-programming our subconscious mind has several benefits and we start developing a strong sense of self-awareness. We are now in control and any negatives, such as 'feel good' and 'what the hell' moments are acted upon before they get out of hand.

Once we are in control, we experience the following signs of progress that we should become familiar with:

- An increase in awareness of our food consumption
- We believe that we are in control of our food intake
- We begin listening to our body and only eating when we are hungry
- We can now say no, or stop eating our meal when we have had enough
- Food is now a pleasure again and not driven by negative emotions
- We are not self-sabotaging or using excuses for breaking the diet
- Temptations, such as supermarket promotions, or restaurant portion sizes, will not play a major part in our food choices.

In short, we'll know when changes are taking place in our subconscious mind because we will notice a shift in both our inner and outer being. The positive signs are usually easy to identify.

Professional help (habit vs addiction)

A question that is regularly asked by professionals is whether obesity is a habit or a form of addiction? A habit is like having an addiction, as we are repeating the same procedure on a regular basis. Typically, addiction can result from an established habit.

However, the rationale is different, and it comes down to the degree of dependence. An addiction can be a well-established psychological need (i.e. an excessive craving) whilst a habit is driven by routine (i.e. having a meal). The difference is that if we miss a meal, it does not turn into a major disruption in our lives and we won't obsessively think about it.

Addictions come in various forms but are typically associated with excessive drug use or smoking. When addiction starts affecting our relationships, job, or health, then professional intervention is recommended. Research has shown that our addictions are the result of several psychosocial factors [36] and may have originated from trauma experienced in our early years. [37] As most of us don't have an addiction to food, the scope of this book does not cover this specialist subject.

If we decide that you may require additional support, as you may have an addiction to food, then consider approaching a professional who specialises in this area. If you discuss, and highlight, our rationale and motivation when it comes to food, they would be able to offer solutions to the underlying issues.

Looking for partner support

If two people are both on the Rehab Weight Loss Plan, then this presents a good opportunity to support each other by providing positive, reassuring encouragement. When presented with a food selection that appears to be greater than we want, then we could discuss what options are best and consider sharing. Sharing a meal is a perfect way of reducing our overall mouthfuls.

Our partner should have read the book to get some understanding of the underlying principles and how to rehab our subconscious mind so that they are in tune with your reduction objectives. Their comments and encouragement need to be positive when we are achieving your objectives and reducing your daily mouthfuls.

Even when we lose track and start overeating, eating more than our baseline consumption, our partner's comments should be positive to a point where we feel some guilt for exceeding our daily food reduction targets.

Summary:
- Meditation is a recognised method of changing established habits for good
- Meditation can help establish a positive, supporting message
- Will help develop a strong sense of self-awareness
- Seek professional advice if you may have an addiction to food
- Partner support will help you achieve your objectives

10. CREATE A FOOD CONSUMPTION BASELINE (Step 3)

Step three of The Rehab Weight Loss Plan:

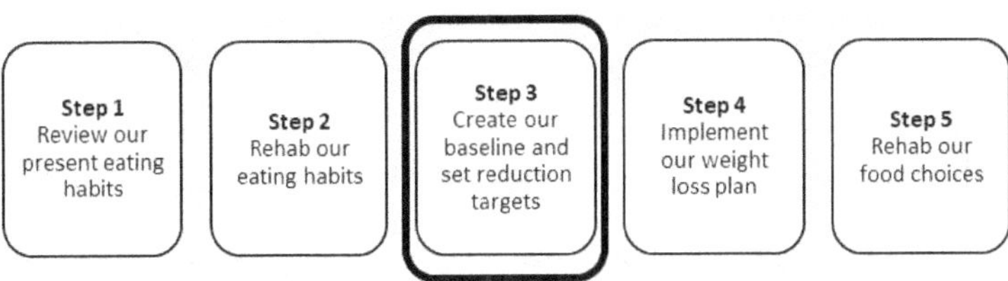

Most people want to feel that they have control of all aspects of their life, whether it is job security, financial issues, or bringing up children. It goes without saying that food, the thing that keeps us alive and gives us so much pleasure, should be on our agenda and one of the aspects that we want to control. Unfortunately, for most of us, our meals have become a non-essential part of our lives, which we have limited control over.

For most of us, our parents never taught us about food control and how much is enough to maintain our body weight. What we think is normal may not be, however, as we have never been told, how are we expected to know? Furthermore, a large part of our food intake has been controlled by third parties (e.g. supermarkets, restaurants) and we have had limited say in the amount of food they are serving us.

One of the main reasons why common diets fail is that our current consumption has never been monitored or recorded. When going on the latest recommended diet, we may in fact be increasing our average daily food consumption. Whilst I was on the Atkin's diet, I constantly felt that I was eating more than my usual daily consumption.

At this point, it is worth noting several well-known management quotes:

…. 'we can't manage what we can't measure'

…. 'we can't save anything (e.g. money) if we have not measured it before'

…. 'we can't compare something that we have never measured'

Simply put, to be a successful manager of a company or a department, we need to have some background history based on reliable facts or data, so we can compare our performance. In this instance, we need to know what our previous food consumption or mouthfuls were, otherwise we will never know how much to reduce our future food intake to lose weight.

Having this data, we can now prepare a plan to help us reduce our consumption. Having a simple weight loss plan will eliminate the feeling of helplessness and the 'what the hell, let's just do it' moments that we experience when we fail to stay on a diet. If we don't have a plan in place to reduce our intake, we are unlikely to lose any weight.

To get some understanding of our food intake, our first objective is to identify what our food consumption baseline is, how many mouthfuls are entering our body during a meal or day. Once we have taken the time to create our food consumption baseline, we will start feeling in control of our eating habits, perhaps for the first time in our lives.

Creating our food consumption baseline

Creating our food consumption baseline is done by counting how many mouthfuls of food we are consuming when eating a single portion of food, a meal, or the total at each sitting (e.g. supper).

There are two main reasons for counting our mouthfuls:

- **Break from our autopilot eating mode:** Generally, when we are counting, we need to concentrate, we are in a conscious state of mind. This will help prevent us from eating in autopilot mode, when we have limited control of the amount of food entering our bodies.
- **Make us more aware of our food intake:** Once we start monitoring how many mouthfuls are entering our mouth at any one time, we will start to understand the following: What our food intake is, so we know how many mouthfuls we must reduce by to lose weight. How

much we have been overeating in the past and the main reason why we are overweight. With time, we will know how many mouthfuls we need to maintain our ideal body weight.

The main aim of this counting exercise is to help us break away from autopilot mode and become more mindful of what we are eating, creating a new 'healthy' habit. Rather than just relying on our subconscious mind to get us through the meal, not thinking about what we are eating.

What meals do we monitor?

These are arranged into two types of meals and consist of:

- **Our main meals:** Consisting of planned meals such as breakfast, lunch and dinner
- **In-between meals:** Consist of our 'in-between' meals, our snacks that we have. You may find that most of our mouthfuls may be coming from snack consumption, food leftovers, chocolate bars, crisps, fruit, etc

Table 1: Types of meals to monitor and record

Meals	Examples
Breakfast	Besides your main meal, to also include all cereals, pieces of toast and fruit
Lunch	Besides your main meal, to also include all add-ons (cheese, sauces) and extras such as packets of crisps, chocolate bars and fruits
Supper / Dinner	Besides your main meal, to also include your starters and deserts, and add-ons such as portions of bread.
In-between meals	Record all food left-overs, fruits, packets of crisps, nuts and chocolate bars
Restaurants and add-ons	Besides your main meal, to also include starters and deserts, and add-ons such as side portions of bread

How do we record our number of mouthfuls?

To record the number of mouthfuls we can either do this mentally or on a piece of paper. This can be a simple stroke of a pencil. At the end of the day, we then add-up our totals, for future reference.

We do recommend that you initially record your mouthfuls on a piece of paper, for future reference. If you don't record this data then there will be a tendency to forget these details, intentionally or not. The aim is to look at the bigger picture, to gain awareness of our food consumption and eating habits. Below is an example of how to create your food consumption baseline.

Table 2: An example of how to record your food consumption baseline.

MY FOOD CONSUMPTION BASELINE			
Meal	Food type	Number of mouthfuls	Total
Breakfast	Full English breakfast - 2*eggs,2* bacon, 2* sausage, mushroom, beans and 2* toast	‖‖‖ ‖‖‖ ‖‖‖ ‖‖‖	18
Snacks	Coffee and a chocolate biscuit	‖‖‖ ‖‖‖	8
Lunch	Cheese burger & portion chips	‖‖‖ ‖‖‖ ‖‖‖ ‖‖‖	20
Snacks	Packet of crisps & Mars bar	‖‖‖ ‖‖‖	8
Snacks	2* beers and 3* helpings of nuts	‖‖‖ ‖‖‖	10
Supper	Spaghetti bolognaise, Garlic bread	‖‖‖ ‖‖‖ ‖‖‖ ‖‖‖ ‖‖‖ ‖‖‖	30
Desert	Apple pie & 1 scope ice-cream	‖‖‖ ‖‖‖ ‖‖‖	12
		MY TOTAL FOR THE DAY	106

It is highly recommended that you record the mouthfuls of your regular meals. Typically, most people have five to seven comfort meals that they eat, on a regular basis, and these must be recorded.

The recording of your baseline will also highlight where most of your consumption is taking place and where to prioritise your time and effort. For example, you may find that your weekend consumption is greater than during the week, as you are eating too many snacks. Now that you are aware of this fact, the obvious solution would be to be either avoid these snacks or reduce your mouthfuls during this period.

Once your food consumption baseline has been established for all your favourite meals, try and visualise your meals by dividing your plate into sections, each section being one mouthful. With time, your mind will recognise if the portions of food that you are about to eat is a 10, 15, or 20 mouthful meal.

My experience:

When I started recording my food baseline consumption, I was surprised to find that I was regularly having 30 to 50 mouthfuls in one meal. When I was going out to a restaurant, I could easily have 80 to 100 mouthfuls in one sitting. Typically, when I was at home and cooking for myself, I was having around 120 to 125 mouthfuls on an average day. On holidays, where we all tend to gain weight, my mouthfuls increased to 130 to 150 per day.

These daily recorded totals all seemed too much for me, however, I had never been told what is normal. It was only when I started constantly recording over 100 mouthfuls daily, did I realise that this was not right. There appeared to be some psychological barrier when I approached 100 mouthfuls and it suggested that I was eating too much.

Although I was constantly trying to eat 'healthy' foods and meals, I was eating too many mouthfuls, without knowing. When I broke down my mouthfuls into my main meals (i.e. breakfast, lunch and supper) and in-between meals (snacks), I discovered that most of my daily consumption was taken up eating snacks (e.g. nuts, fruit crisps, chocolate bars, left-overs in the fridge, etc).

During the week, it appeared that I was in control of my food consumption, however, at weekends I was out of control and overindulging on food and alcohol.

In summary:
- We need to create a food consumption baseline as we have never quantified how much food we consume
- Counting our mouthfuls will help us break from our autopilot mode
- Counting our mouthfuls will make us become more aware of our food intake
- All our favourite meals and in-between meals (e.g. snacks) need to be recorded
- This may take one to two weeks, depending on how many different types of meals we normally eat
- It is recommended that we record our mouthfuls on a piece of paper for future reference.

11. HOW MANY MOUTHFULS ARE ENOUGH? (Step 3)

Having successfully monitored our number of mouthfuls and recorded our food consumption baseline, we can now set our reduction targets to reduce the number of mouthfuls entering our body, to help us lose weight.

How many mouthfuls are enough?

Documented research has shown that the recommended daily food allowance for an average adult man is 2500 kcal, to maintain his weight, and 2000 kcal to start experiencing weight loss. An average adult woman needs 2000 kcal, to maintain her weight, and 1500 kcal to start experiencing weight loss. [38]

These recommended daily calorie intakes will depend on your physical height, age, shape, the amount of daily exercise and how active your metabolism is. These recommended daily food allowances do not necessarily apply to all adults and should be a rough guide only.

Understanding the food amount and related calorie content, of one mouthful, is almost impossible to calculate as there are several factors that we need to take into consideration:

- **The type of food:** The calorific value of foods varies significantly. For the same sized mouthful, a bite from a Mars bar can be as much as 45 kcal, whilst a slice of ham can be around 10 kcal
- **Calculating the daily average value:** During a typical day, we may be eating a range of foods, some with higher and others with lower-calorie values. We, therefore, need to take the average calories per mouthful across the entire day
- **Your mouthful size:** Not all our mouthfuls will be 100% full when eating and there may be a difference in the size of our mouths

When we apply any mathematical calculation that includes more than three variables, such as the above, the result is not perfect. Research suggests that the number of calories is around 17 per mouthful for an adult. [39]

When we use an average of 20 kcal per mouthful, for convenience, the benchmark table below will give us an indication of the number of mouthfuls we need to satisfy our daily recommended allowance. The table will also highlight how many mouthfuls we need to lose weight.

Note: We can't scientifically confirm that the average content of a mouthful of food is 20 kcal and there appears to be limited research on the subject. This average figure should be used as an estimated guide.

Table 3: Mouthful benchmark table reference

MOUTHFUL BENCHMARK TABLE		
	Man (kcal)	Women (kcal)
To maintain your weight		
Recommended Calories to maintain your weight/day	2500	2000
Average calories per mouthfuls	20	20
Mouthfuls to maintain your weight /day	**125**	**100**
Recommended calories to lose weight		
Recommended Calories to reduce your weight/day	2000	1500
Average calories per mouthfuls	20	20
Mouthfuls to reduce your weight /day	**100**	**75**
To reduce our calories further		
If we set a Calorie target /day	1500	1000
Average calories per mouthfuls	20	20
Mouthfuls to further reduce your weight /day	**75**	**50**

When referring to the above table, we can see that to meet the recommended calorie intake to maintain our body weight, it is estimated that we need around 125 mouthfuls for a man and 100 mouthfuls for women.

If your daily mouthfuls have been constantly exceeding 125 mouthfuls for a man, and 100 for a woman, it suggests that you have been overeating and the main reason you are overweight.

After the first week, having recorded your mouthful baseline consumption, you should be able to do some simple comparisons to see how your daily consumption compares with the above table. This should be used as a rough benchmark to give you an indication of where you are and help you prepare your future food reduction targets.

Food consumption comparison

People typically tend to want to compare their progress with third-party comparisons, such as benchmarks. However, as there are so many variables when it comes to calculating the value of your food calorie intake per mouthful, we need to be more realistic when comparing.

During the monitoring stage, when recording our mouthfuls, it should be a voyage of discovery to make us more aware of our food intake and what the overall consumption is on average. It will also help us stop eating in autopilot mode and promote new, good habits.

Our objective at this stage is to determine what our food consumption baseline is, our daily mouthfuls. It is more important that we enjoy our food and not become too obsessed with comparing with external targets.

Summary
- It is important to understand our food intake, what our daily total mouthfuls are
- When using 20 kcal per mouthful, as an average, this will give us an indication of our daily calorie consumption
- Counting our mouthfuls at meals will help us stop eating in autopilot
- This will give us an idea of how much we are consuming on an average day
- This will give us an indication of how much we may have been overeating in the past
- Now we have quantified our daily mouthfuls, we can easily regulate our food intake to lose weight

12. SETTING MOUTHFUL REDUCTION TARGETS (Step 3)

Setting some form of target in life, whether it is for self-improvement or career goals, gives us a purpose and a reason to achieve something fulfilling. Once we have achieved a milestone, we typically experience a positive warm feeling of achievement. This should be extended to our weight loss plan and setting mouthful reduction targets will keep us motivated to make sure our objectives are achieved.

Setting food intake reduction targets

Having monitored and recorded our food consumption baseline, the number of mouthfuls that we have for all our meals, we can now set our mouthful reduction targets for each meal, or for the day.

For example, if we are having over 20 to 30 mouthfuls for a single meal (e.g. lunch) then consider reducing by 5 mouthfuls, then a week later, consider reducing by another 5 mouthfuls.

If we are having over 40 to 50 mouthfuls for a single meal (e.g. supper) then consider reducing by 10 mouthfuls, then a week later, consider reducing by another 5 mouthfuls.

Overall, if we aim to reduce each meal by 5 to 10 mouthfuls, we would have a potential reduction in our total daily mouthful intake of food of around 20 to 25%. This is a good, simple starting point for our mouthful reduction plan.

Table 4: An example how to set targets to reduce our mouthfuls.

MOUTHFUL REDUCTION TARGETS			
Meal type	Present mouthfuls	New target	% Consumption saving
Breakfast	25	20	20%
Lunch	30	20	33%
Supper	50	40	20%
In-between meals	20	10	50%
Total	**125**	**90**	**28%**

In the above example, we have reduced our overall total by 35 mouthfuls for the day, resulting in a reduction of 28% less food going into our body. With a regular reduction in our daily food intake, we will soon experience the feeling of weight loss and our weighing scales will confirm this.

For those who are consistently having more than 100 mouthfuls per day, consider setting a target of eating no more than 100 mouthfuls per day. Consider using this daily target as an imaginary psychological barrier that we need to break though. This 'breaking' of this imaginary barrier will spur us on and help us control our daily food intake. Once we have achieved this on a regular basis, then consider lowering the barrier to a new, lower target, say 90 mouthfuls per day.

Once we are regularly reducing the number of mouthfuls of favourite food entering our mouth each day, and we see that this is no major sacrifice, we will start feeling in control and motivated to stay on our weight loss plan.

Realistic food reduction targets

People who want to change their lifestyle typically let their enthusiasm overtake them and they tend to 'dive' into their new venture and this leads to failure, especially if the desired results (loss of weight) don't happen overnight. In this case, reducing our mouthful intake by a significant amount, say 40 to 50%, may make us feel deprived of our favourite foods and we may feel hungry resulting in us going back to our 'old ways'.

Alternatively, we could 'by-pass' the system by setting modest daily reductions, say one to two mouthfuls, however the only person we are fooling will be ourselves. Remember that we don't usually taste our food after the first five mouthfuls, so setting aggressive reduction targets should not be a challenge. We are in the process of changing a lifetime habit which will be a challenge for us, especially if we always considered our food to be a treat. We will be more likely to agree with realistic food intake target that are achievable.

Research has shown that we can expect to lose 1.0 to 2.0 pound (0.5 to 1.0 kg) per week, [40] that is, if we are constantly keeping our daily average calories below 2000 kcal for a man, and 1500 kcal for a woman. When setting our reduction targets, we need to aim to reduce our overall calorie intake by around 500 kcal each day, around 3500 kcal in total for the week, if we want to lose 1.0 (0.5kg). Reducing our overall daily food intake by, say 20 to 30 mouthfuls, will ensure that our reduction in total calories will be around 3500 kcal at the end of the week, which will not be a great sacrifice for us.

Realistic daily food reduction targets are a good start, and we must appreciate that this is not a competition to see how much weight we can lose in the shortest period. We are wanting to change a well-established habit, rather than experience another short-term weight loss.

Take one day at a time and see each target that we complete as an achievement. Our new 'less is good' habits will form, which will change our future eating habits for good and this will improve our chances of achieving our weight loss goals.

My experience:

As I had never quantified how many mouthfuls, I was consuming at any one time, I was not aware of what was normal or how much I could reduce my mouthfuls for each meal. My main concern was that I may feel hungry, which was driven by my beliefs that I needed three meals per day to survive.

Initially, my targets were conservative, I aimed for a reduction of 5 mouthfuls per meal, for the first week. I then further reduced my food intake by another 5 mouthfuls per meal. Over time, I have managed to reduce my overall daily food intake to around 50 to 70 mouthfuls per day, without feeling hungry and any adverse effect on my overall health. If anything, I have experienced a boost in my energy levels and wellbeing.

Summary:
- Knowing our food consumption baseline, we can now implement our reduction targets
- We need to set a mouthful reduction target for each meal
- The reduction targets must be realistic
- We should aim for a reduction target of 20 to 30 mouthfuls daily (20 to 30% saving in consumption)
- Overall, we should aim for a daily reduction of 500 kcal, around 3500 kcal per week, to start experiencing weight loss

13. IMPLEMENT OUR WEIGHT LOSS PLAN (Step 4)

Step four of the Rehab Weight Loss Plan:

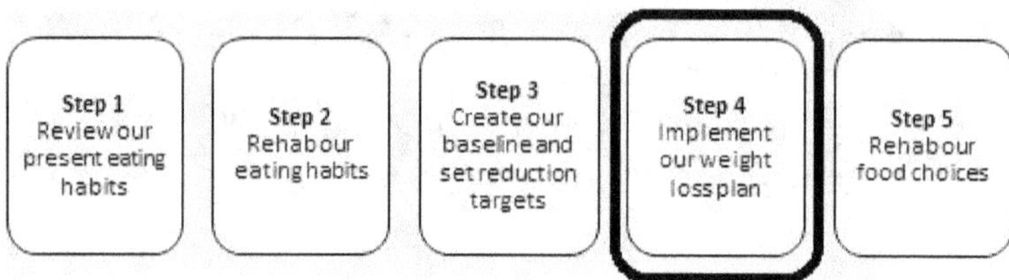

Now that we know our food consumption baseline, and we have set our reduction targets, we need to implement our weight loss plan. There are several recognised methods, which most of us should be familiar with, are highlighted below.

Have a smaller meal portion.

When having an 'assembled' type meal, that consists of protein (e.g. cooked meat, chicken) and vegetables (e.g. potatoes, carrots), always consider eating a smaller-sized portion. For roast meat meals, if there are three pieces of meat, consider removing one piece from our plate.

Alternatively, eat all our meat portions, as they have good protein content, and then reduce our add-on portions, such as potatoes and vegetables. In most cases, we tend to 'load' up our plates with starchy foods (e.g. potatoes, rice) which we can easily reduce as, after a few mouthfuls, we stop tasting these foods as we have eaten them on numerous occasions.

When ordering meals in a restaurant, given the choice between having a larger or smaller food portion (e.g. a steak), we should always consider ordering a smaller-sized portion. When add-ons come with the meal, we should always eat a smaller portion than what is on the plate (i.e. only eat half a portion of rice).

Stop when you have reached your mouthful target

When we are in a restaurant, where the food is prepared from a recipe, (e.g. Indian, Chinese or Italian) when we have no, or limited, control of the portion size that they are serving us. We need to reduce our food intake, the number of mouthfuls entering our body.

Consider only eating up to your pre-set target, say 10 mouthfuls, then stop. In these scenarios, you should challenge the need for a large portion by using the Rehab 'less is good' habit-change strategy.

Alternatively, another option would be to separate your plate of food into quarters, with your knife and fork, then don't eat one of the quarters. This simple routine will make sure that you stop eating, or clearing, all the food on the plate.

Order an alternative smaller-sized meal portion

Some of us would confirm that most of our food choices are chosen by size. Given the choice between having a meal comprising a larger food portion (e.g. a large pasta dish), than one that is smaller (e.g. a fish dish), we will tend to order the bigger portion, especially if it is roughly the same cost.

Our food choice has nothing to do with us being hungry as it was our well-established 'more is good' habits influencing our decision. Going to a restaurant has always been a treat, a special occasion, that our parents gave us for good behaviour.

When we are presented with this scenario, our food choice should be influenced by the taste sensation, not our 'more is good' habit. Always consider a smaller food portion as this will help create our new 'less is good' eating habit.

The table below highlights the number of mouthfuls that we typically consume when having our usual meals. The right-side highlights how we can reduce our portion sizes.

Table 5: Replacing large for smaller-sized meals: [41]

LARGER FOR SMALLER MEAL TYPES					
Existing meal			**Consider changing for**		
	kcal	Mouthfuls		kcal	Mouthfuls
BREAKFAST					
Full English breakfast - 2*eggs,2* bacon, 2* sausage, mushroom, black pudding, beans and 2* toast	1400	40 to 50	Small English breakfast - 1*egg, 1*bacon, 1*sausage, mushroom, beans	460	10 to 15
			Eggs Benedict - 1*egg, ham and sauce	450	10 to 15
			One fried egg and bacon in a roll	400	10 to 15
Average English breakfast - 2*eggs, 2*bacon slices, 2*toast	860	30 to 40	Scrambled eggs, smoked salmon, on toast - 1*eggs	540	10 to 15
Eggs Benedict - 2*eggs, ham, 2* buns, and sauce	600	20 to 30	Scrambled 1*egg, bacon wrap	530	8 to 10
			Scrambled 1*egg on toast	360	8 to 10
American style pancakes and maple syrup	720	20 to 30	Mashed avocado on toast	410	8 to 10
			Beans on toast	480	8 to 10
			Mini style pancakes and syrup	430	8 to 10
BURGER MEALS					
Beef Burger (6 oz) and chips - with cheese, BBQ sauce.	1320	40 to 50	Smaller burger (3.7 oz) - with cheese, BBQ sauce - (no chips)	550	10 to 12
Portion of chips (560 kcal)					
Grilled chicken burger with bacon and salad (530)	1090	30 to 35	Chicken burger with salad (no chips)	440	10 to 12
Portion of chips (560 kcal)			Vegetable burger (no chips)	500	10 to 12
PIZZA MEALS					
Margareta pizza (12 inch)	1060	30 to 40	Only eat half of the pizza (3 slices)	650	10 to 12
Pepperoni Pizza (12 inch)	1300				
Roasted vegetable pizza (12 inch)	900		Only eat 2 pizza slices and a salad	400	8 to 10
Spicy meat feast (12 inch)	1340				
Garlic bread (4 slices)	200	10 to 12	Garlic bread (1-2 slices)	100	3 to 4
ITALIAN MEALS					
Spaghetti Bolognese	720	20 to 30	Reduce by 5 mouthfuls to start. Reduce pasta portion size.	500	10 to 12
Beef Lasagne (no chips)	750	20 to 30			
Vegetable lasagne	600	20 to 30			
Garlic pizza bread – large	890	8 to 10	Share with others	440	3 to 4

INDIAN CURRY MEALS					
	kcal	Mouthfuls		kcal	Mouthfuls
Chicken Jalfrezi curry (410 kcal)	890	30 to 40	Reduce by 5 mouthfuls to start. Replace Naan bread for chapatti and reduce rice portion. Avoid starters (poppadum, pickle tray)	600	15 to 20
Rice, Naan bread and poppadum's (480 kcal)					
Chicken Korma curry (520 kcal)	1000	30 to 40			
Rice, Naan bread and poppadum's (480 kcal)					
Lamb Rogan Josh Curry (580 kcal)	1060	30 to 40			
Rice, Naan bread and poppadum's (480 kcal)					
Sweet potato, chickpea curry and rice (350 kcal)	830	20 to 30			
Rice, Naan bread and poppadums' (480 kcal)					
Samosa and onion bhaji snacks	405	4 to 6	Share with others	150	2 to 3

PROTEIN / MEAT TYPE MEALS					
8 oz Beef sirloin steak (600 kcal)	1060	20 to 30	5 oz Skinny Sirloin steak with salad. Reduce portion size of chips	650	10 to 12
Portion of chips (560 kcal)					
12 oz Rump steak	750	16 to 18			
Mixed grill - with pork lion, sausage, egg and onion rings	870	25 to 28			

COMMON MEALS					
Beef Cottage pie with chips	1010	20 to 25	Beef Cottage pie (small) with salad	650	10 to 12
Beef Chilli with rice	770	20 to 25	Beef Chilli with salad, or reduce rice portion	600	10 to 12
Fish and chips - large (1230 kcal)	1670	30 to 40	Small fish and reduce portion of chips. No bread	840	10 to 12
Two slices of bread (440 kcal)					
Scampi and chips	900	18 to 20	Chicken salad, bacon and avocado	430	10 to 12
BBQ pork ribs - full rack	1100	18 to 20	BBQ pork ribs - half rack	600	10 to 12
Southern fried chicken strips (5 pieces)	533	18 to 20	Southern fried chicken strips (3 pieces)	280	8 to 10
Gammon Steak (400 grams), egg and chips	900	18 to 20	Reduce in size and half of chips	500	8 to 10

CHINESE MEALS					
Beef Chow Mein	860	15 to 20	Reduce by 5 mouthfuls to start.	470	8 to 12
Sweet & Sour Pork (440 kcal)	756	15 to 20	Reduce by 5 mouthfuls to start. Reduce rice portion size.	380	8 to 12
Fried rice (316 kcal)					
Beef in black bean sauce (410 kcal)	654	15 to 20	Reduce by 5 mouthfuls to start. Reduce noddle portion size.	360	8 to 12
Noodles (244 kcal)					

On the left-side of the above table gives us an indication of how many mouthfuls there are in a typical meal. Replacing these meals, for smaller-sized portions containing reduced mouthfuls, on the right, will lower our overall calorie content, by as much as half.

There is no reason why we can't eat our favourite foods that we regularly have. We can still order our regular meals on the left-side; however, we will need to stop eating once we have reached our mouthful reduction target for the day. We will still experience the same rationale for having the meal (e.g. the taste and smell sensation) and the 'feel good' moment.

To avoid any temptation, always consider ordering the smaller portions, as food that is not on our plate does not become a temptation for us to 'clear' the plate. Alternatively, consider sharing the food portion with your partner.

With time, we should be able to visualise what our food portion size should be and how many mouthfuls it will take to finish. We will soon be able to recognise which meals are significantly larger in portion size. With this basic information, you should now be able to start reducing your mouthfuls on a regular basis, introducing our 'less is good' eating habit.

In-between meals (snacks) on your weight loss plan

Besides reducing our mouthfuls for our main meals, we also need to consider our 'in-between' meals, our snacks. Some snacks are a treat, a 'feel good' moment of memories of our childhood, and the temptation to snack may be difficult to give up completely.

There are two types of snacks; one is of high-carbohydrates foods such as chocolate, crisps, biscuits, sandwiches, pizza slices, pastry, or cakes. The other is the healthier type and these consist of fruit, vegetables, nuts, leftover food or a small yogurt pot or cereal.

The table below shows a comparison of snack types per 100-grams. As food portions come in all shapes and sizes, when comparing foods, we should always relate the calories, and contents, to a fixed, common value (i.e. 100 grams).

Table 6: Calorie Content of popular Snacks per 100 grams [42]

CALORIE CONTENT OF SNACKS per 100 grams (3,5 oz)					
Snacks with HIGH Calories			Alternative with LOW calories		
Food type	Mouthfuls	kcal	Food type	Mouthfuls	kcal
Nuts mixed - unsalted	4 to 6	530	Ham - boiled	4 to 6	105
Crisps - salted	4 to 6	524	Prawns	4 to 6	98
Sausage roll	4 to 6	507	Cottage cheese	4 to 6	66
Kit Kat chunky	4 to 6	490	Apple	4 to 6	42
Mars bar	4 to 6	440	Satsuma	4 to 6	42
Cream crackers	4 to 6	440	Kiwi	4 to 6	42
Cheese Cheddar	4 to 6	410	Orange	4 to 6	36
Popcorn - salted	4 to 6	395	Peach	4 to 6	30
Toffee bar	4 to 6	388	Strawberries	4 to 6	25
Pork pie	4 to 6	328	Yogurt natural	4 to 6	60
Garlic pizza bread	4 to 6	340	Melon	4 to 6	16

Referring to the table, we can see that most of the snacks on the left-side are processed foods, such as pies, chocolate, crisps and have higher calories per 100 grams than alternatives, such as fruits and yogurts. If we snack on healthier foods, on the right of the table, it will help us lose weight.

Given the choice of one pork pie (328 kcal) or one peach (30 kcal), we can see that the total number of mouthfuls, per item, would be roughly the same (4 to 6 mouthfuls), but we would have a saving of around 300 calories. The good news is that one peach would give you the same 'filling' sensation as a pork pie and most people would not eat ten peaches in a row. This highlights the importance of eating low-calorie food on the right-side of the table.

Furthermore, our choice should be based on nutritional value as well. The average-sized Mars bar has 240 kcal. We could, as a substitute, have one apple (40 kcal), with the same number of mouthfuls (4 to 6) and we would have a saving of around 300 calories. The main difference is that the Mars bar has limited nutritional content. We are now saving on calories as well as improving the quality of food we are eating.

However, it should be noted that this table highlights the calorie content per 100 grams. There are some snacks on the left that are considered good for us, such as nuts and cheese, which have proven nutritional benefits. Typically, a portion of nuts is around 30 grams (200 kcal) and a slice of cheese is around 25 grams (100 kcal). This is no reason why we can't eat these snacks if they are in moderation.

When we are on a diet, we tend to think that we are in control of our mouthfuls (calories), during our main meals. However, if we are eating in-between meals (snacks), consisting of 30 to 40 mouthfuls during the day, then we are adding a significant number of extra calories into our bodies. The mouthful consumption of all snacks must be included in Step three when creating your food consumption baseline. We need to treat our in-between meals (snacks) the same as our main meals.

On the Rehab Weight Loss Plan, or any other diet, these unhealthy processed snacks, on the left-side of the table, should always be avoided as, besides the high-calorie content, they can also have excessive sugar and salt content. The golden rule is we should avoid all processed foods and substitute for whole or raw food ingredients where possible.

Fig 4: Something to think about, chocolate muffin (250 kcal) vs apple (70 kcal)

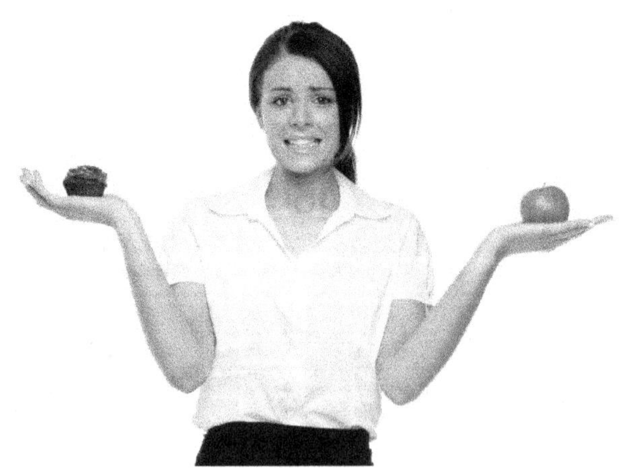

Further tips to help us reduce our number of mouthfuls during the day:

Brunch instead of breakfast

Breakfast is one of our meals where we don't put much thought into the process and is a well-established habit. We wake up and then eat our breakfast, in autopilot, not having had time to think if we need the meal or not. In most cases, our biggest meal of the day is supper, which we had the previous evening. If we have been sleeping overnight, with minimal physical activity, why then do we need to have a big breakfast?

It's about having another 'feel good' moment as our parents have constantly reassured us that 'breakfast is the most important meal of the day'. Most will confirm that this statement is not necessarily true and another misbelief that we have inherited from our childhood.

In my childhood, I typically started most breakfasts with a bowl of cereal. As my mother was allowing me to fill up my bowl with cereal and milk, I was constantly having a greater portion than needed. In most instances, having finished the contents of my first helping, and as the box of cereal and the milk were still on the table, I would automatically add another helping to the bowl and then proceed to finish that portion.

If my mother had only given me a pre-filled bowl, with an average portion of cereal and milk, and no second helpings, I would have accepted this fact, like every other meal that she had prepared for me. Now, on most mornings, I seldom have breakfast. This suggests that, previously, this meal was driven out of a well-established habit that had nothing to do with hunger.

If you consider having brunch, a combination of breakfast and lunch consumed in mid-morning, it is an excellent way of reducing your daily mouthfuls. As we are having two meals at once, whilst only consuming the number of mouthfuls for one meal, this allows us to reduce our overall total for the day, potentially a 20 to 30% reduction in mouthfuls and calories.

Avoiding breakfast completely or having a small bite to eat (a banana or a small yogurt pot) with a cup of coffee will, with time, become a good habit as we are now listening to our engine and only eating when we need to. This will also help achieve our overall daily mouthful targets on our weight loss plan.

Eating hot instead of cold food

In my experience, having a hot, nutritious cooked meal is tastier and will satisfy my hunger more than a cold meal, especially during the winter. This may be because a large part of our taste sensation involves smell, so hot food provides positive support when it comes to its selection. [43]

On a cold day, given the choice of having a small, hot lasagne (5 to 8 mouthfuls) or a cold chicken salad (10 to 14 mouthfuls), you should consider having the hot meal as there are less mouthfuls and it will give you more of taste satisfaction and a filling sensation. Although the salad may have less calories per grams, depending on how many mouthfuls of salad you have, you could be eating the same number of calories without knowing. In most cities, there are now many food outlets offering a range of good, hot meals and most have fewer than 500 calories.

It should be noted that, when in a hot country, this option may work the other way around with us wanting a cold meal, a salad, or similar.

Storing your mouthfuls for later

If you know that you are going out later, to a favourite restaurant, then you should consider storing or 'banking' mouthfuls. So, instead of having ten mouthfuls for both breakfast and lunch, consider having five mouthfuls for each meal, or have brunch instead.

That will give you a credit of ten extra mouthfuls that you can have when sitting down for your restaurant meal. The theory is that we are now beginning to listen to our bodies, and we are not just eating to satisfy our habit. This will help us not exceed our daily targets.

Serving smaller portion sizes

When preparing meals for the family, you should be able to visualise the food portion sizes. Serving smaller food portions means we are not overeating, and we are reducing our waste as we are not throwing away leftovers. This will avoid any temptation to finish the last few mouthfuls. Food that is not served, or seen on our plate, should not be wasted and this will develop a good habit.

A further consideration is to serve our food on smaller-sized plates. Over the past decade, we have tended to purchase larger-sized plates which has led to more food being served on our plate, either intentionally or not.

Eating more slowly

Research has shown that eating our meals more slowly, keeping our bites of food longer in our mouth, can help us reduce our consumption of food. [44] Eating more slowly allows the receptors in the stomach to travel to the brain to tell us when we are satisfied, and this will hopefully reduce our food intake. However, if we are constantly eating in autopilot mode, I am not sure if this will help us reduce our mouthfuls.

Most of us tend to eat our meals too quickly. So, eating our meals more slowly will make us appreciate our food and it is recommended and that we extend the duration of our meals where possible.

Revisiting your original Food Consumption Baseline

Now that we are regularly reducing our mouthfuls at each meal, it is worth considering recording how many mouthfuls we are consuming as this allows us an opportunity to compare. This simple recording of our new mouthful targets against our 'old' consumption (our baseline), will give us an understanding of our progress.

This will highlight the fact that we can reduce our mouthfuls, our food intake, without feeling any major disruption to our usual consumption. This will prove that your new 'less is good' habit is not a great sacrifice and will give us the motivation to carry on.

Table 7: Comparing your recorded mouthfuls for your favourite foods

<table>
<thead>
<tr><th colspan="6" align="center">MY FOOD CONSUMPTION BASELINE</th></tr>
<tr><th>Food type</th><th>Number of mouthfuls</th><th>Total</th><th>My new mouthfuls</th><th>Total</th><th>Comment</th></tr>
</thead>
<tbody>
<tr><td>Full English breakfast - 2*eggs,2* bacon, 2* sausage, mushroom, beans and 2* toast</td><td>卌 卌 卌 卌</td><td>20</td><td>卌 卌</td><td>10</td><td>Now only have 1*egg, 1*slice bacon, no beans or toast</td></tr>
<tr><td>Large Cheese burger (3 patty) & large portion of fries & coke</td><td>卌 卌 卌 III</td><td>18</td><td>卌 卌</td><td>10</td><td>Only order small burger. Reduced fries portion by half. Order low-calorie coke option</td></tr>
<tr><td>Spaghetti bolognaise & Garlic bread</td><td>卌 卌 卌 III</td><td>18</td><td>卌 III</td><td>8</td><td>Only eat half of the meal and take-home. No garlic bread</td></tr>
<tr><td>Steak (12 oz), chips, 2* bread rolls</td><td>卌 卌 卌 II</td><td>17</td><td>卌 卌</td><td>10</td><td>Order small steak portion. Reduced chips portion by half. No bread rolls</td></tr>
<tr><td>Chicken curry, rice, naan bread and pickle tray</td><td>卌 卌 卌 卌 II</td><td>22</td><td>卌 卌 II</td><td>12</td><td>Eat only half of the meal and take-home. No naan bread and pickle tray</td></tr>
<tr><td>Fish and chips. 2* bread slices</td><td>卌 卌 卌 III</td><td>18</td><td>卌 III</td><td>8</td><td>Order small portion. Reduced chips portion by half. No bread</td></tr>
<tr><td>Roast chicken, vegetables & roast potatoes</td><td>卌 卌 卌 II</td><td>17</td><td>卌 卌</td><td>10</td><td>Reduced roasted potato portion by half. No bread</td></tr>
<tr><td>Large 12' meat pizza</td><td>卌 卌 卌 卌 II</td><td>22</td><td>卌 III</td><td>8</td><td>Only had 3 slices and take -home for another meal</td></tr>
<tr><td>Beef chilli, rice & bread roll</td><td>卌 卌 卌 II</td><td>17</td><td>卌 III</td><td>8</td><td>Reduced rice portion by half. No bread</td></tr>
</tbody>
</table>

If we constantly aim for 8 to 12 mouthfuls, for the regular meals that we are eating, including add-ons (i.e. bread), then we don't necessarily have to record our mouthfuls. We would be creating a new 'less is good' habit which will be with us for life. However, to create our new habit we need to repeat the exercise on a regular basis to make it a well-established one.

Summary:

- Always prepare or order a smaller meal portion
- Stop when you have reached your mouthful target
- Consider ordering an alternative meal that has a smaller-sized portion
- Review your consumption of in-between meals (snacks)
- Consider having brunch instead of breakfast or lunch
- Consider eating hot meals instead of cold ones
- Consider 'banking' your mouthfuls of an earlier meal for later
- Eat your meals more slowly to help reduce consumption

- Revisit your food consumption baseline to compare progress
- By constantly reducing our food portions, we will be creating a new 'less is good' habit.

14. REHAB OUR FOOD CHOICES AT HOME (Step 5)

Step five of the Rehab Weight Loss Plan:

The objective of Rehab Weight Loss Plan is to help us change our eating habits and make us more food-aware, by improving our food choices. This book does not come with recommended recipes, food plans, etc. There are hundreds of these types of books on the market highlighting low-calorie meal options and it is not necessary to provide further information on this subject. Furthermore, we believe that once we 'rehab' our food choice habits and become more food-aware, we won't need to purchase the latest cookbook endorsed by a well-known celebrity.

Now that we are constantly challenging our large food portion sizes, by introducing our new 'less is good' habits, we need to review our food choice habits, our rationale for why we choose certain foods over others. Our foods, that we are consuming regularly, maybe high-calorie options with limited nutritional content (e.g. processed foods), however, they are our favourites.

There are two underlying issues: most of our food choices originate from a belief that we have inherited (e.g. cereals are good for you, even though some have a large sugar content), or we have no or limited understanding of the calorie content of our regular meals. As highlighted, research shows that 60% of people in the UK have a limited understanding of their daily calorie consumption. [45]

If we are constantly introducing our new 'less is good' eating habits, this should inevitably start reducing our overall daily food portion sizes. When it comes to food preparation at home, it should become routine that we start reducing the physical size, or weight, of our cooking ingredients.

Introduction

Eating a sensible, balanced diet consisting of protein, vegetables and fruit is the basis for healthy eating and our wellbeing. It can promote growth, development and performance as well as maintain our health for a lifetime. [46] With the increase in obesity and nutrition-related diseases, changing our diet to one that is balanced and healthy is therefore of importance.

Most of our daily meals are cooked and eaten at home. It can be difficult to know what the ideal food portion sizes are, as we may be influenced by our childhood experiences and the media (TV). Furthermore, our meals come in all forms, shapes and portion sizes and it can be a challenge for us to determine which foods have more calories than others.

Eating processed food, high in carbohydrates or trans-fats such as pizza, pies, hot chips, cereals and cakes, are generally considered to have a higher calorie content per 100 grams.

The foods which have a good protein and nutrient content, such as meats, chicken, fish, vegetables and fruits are generally considered better and healthier for us. Typically, these healthy foods have fewer calories per 100 grams. If we want to give our weight loss a boost, then is it worth considering making some alterations to our daily food intake, to include these foods.

With time, whilst on our weight-reduction plan, we will feel the positive momentum from our weight loss and find that we naturally gravitate from high-calorie foods towards more healthy eating options.

Rehab your supermarket shopping habits

In most cases, our visits to the supermarket are now well-established routines. We have standard foods that we look for when we enter a supermarket as we all, typically, have five to seven go-to meals.

To help us become more food aware, to help change our food choice habits, we need to constantly challenge our thought processes when entering our local supermarket. Changing these food choice habits at source, at the supermarket, will mean less temptation for us to eat larger meals when at home.

When entering a supermarket, it is generally recommended that we should be looking for meal ingredients that are:

- High in protein (e.g. meats, chicken, fish)
- Have good nutritional value (e.g. vegetables, salads or fruits)
- Drinks that are nutritious and low-calorie

At all times we should avoid, or limit:

- High carbohydrate food options such as pizza and types of breads
- High-calorie meals with large sugar and salt content, such as desserts, chocolates and biscuits
- High-calorie 'ready-meals' or processed foods types (e.g. pies, pastries, snacks)
- Alcohol and sugary drinks with a high-calorie or sugar content.

The above suggestions are general recommendations, found in most diet books, to help promote healthy foods.

Improve our food choices

To improve our food choices, we need to become more food aware. Most foods come with the nutritional content information on the packaging and this should indicate which foods have low or high calories per 100 grams.

When preparing meals for yourself, or others, we recommend that you consider the following:

- Always look for the calories per 100 grams on the packaging
- Aim for food products with low calories per 100 grams (i.e. 100 to

200 kcal per 100 grams)

- Avoid processed food products, with high calories per 100 grams, having minimal nutritional value with high salt and sugar content
- Where food products have a high calories per 100 grams, consider reducing the portion size, when cooking or serving

When purchasing 'ready-meals', or similar, look for the total calories /serving on the packaging. Any meals with a calorie per serving above 500 kcal should be avoided or consider sharing with a partner or stop eating once your mouthful target has been reached.

Always aim for meals, with add-ons, with a calorie content of around 400 to 500 kcal, that take 8 to 12 mouthfuls to finish.

If we are constantly preparing meals that are low in calories per 100 grams, are smaller in portion size, then fewer calories should be entering our body, our engine. There should be no logical reason why you won't lose weight.

Fig 5: Our goal, when shopping, should be low calorie, high nutrients foods

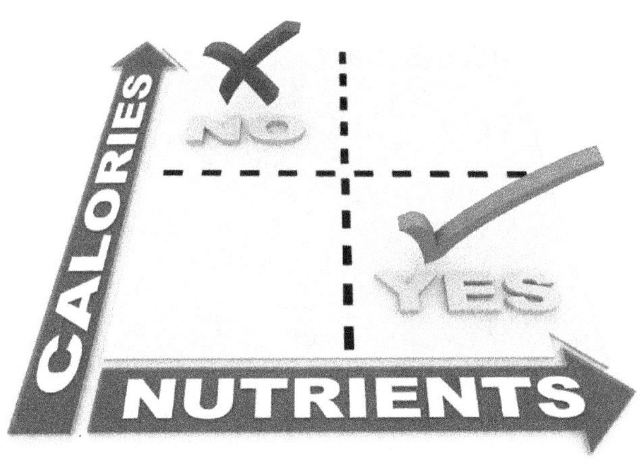

Nutritional information labels

The below nutritional information label highlights the necessity to look out for this information. Referring to the below table, we can see that for a 100 grams portion, there is a calorie content of 93 kcal. However, the whole pack contains 339 kcal, which is far greater. When we then add the 'extras' to our meal (e.g. rice and vegetables), the overall total calories for the meal could be 700 to 800 kcal.

Fig 6: Typical nutritional label of a food product

NUTRITION

When microwaved according to instructions

Typical values	Per 100g	Each pack (366g**)	% RI*	RI* for an average adult
Energy	390kJ / 93kcal	1429kJ / 339kcal	17%	8400kJ / 2000kcal
Fat	2.3g	8.3g	12%	70g
of which saturates	1.1g	4.1g	21%	20g
Carbohydrate	14.0g	51.1g		
of which sugars	1.7g	6.3g	7%	90g
Fibre	1.4g	5.1g		
Protein	3.4g	12.4g		
Salt	0.4g	1.5g	25%	6g

Pack contains 1 serving
*Reference intake of an average adult (8400kJ / 2000kcal)
**When microwaved according to instructions 385g typically weighs 366g

Avoid sales promotions

When we are presented with a sales promotion, a 'more is good' temptation, that could lead to a 'what the hell, let's just do it' moment, we should always consider the following statements:

…. *'these desserts are wasted calories. Why am I buying this?'*

…. *'why am I buying these multi-pack chocolate bars, we will only eat them'*

…. *'this pie has over 400 calories per 100 grams. Why am I buying this?'*

…. *'this treat has over 500 calories per serving. Why am I buying this?'*

…. *'I am not going to be influenced by this pizza sales offer'*

By constantly challenging the need to purchase these items, by using verbal repetition of a positive message, can help re-programme (rehab) our subconscious mind. This will help change our food choice habits for healthy ones, not influenced by third parties.

Preparing meals at home

The table below shows a list of everyday foods, highlighting their calories per 100 grams, so we can compare it with other food types. This provides a useful tool if we want to change high-calorie food with one of lower-calorie content.

Table 8: Calorie content of food types (high calorie) per 100 grams. [47]

CALORIE CONTENT OF FOOD TYPE per 100 grams (3,5 oz)			
Meals with HIGH Calories		**HIGH to MEDIUM Calories**	
Food type	kcal	Food type	kcal
Butter	740	Pork sausage - grilled	290
Margarine	680	French fries - takeaway	290
Peanut Butter nutty	606	Doughnut iced	285
Pork crackling	550	Bacon - grilled	284
Nuts mixed - unsalted	530	Bagel - plain	270
Crisps -salted	524	Omelette with cheese	266
Sausage roll	507	Jam - strawberry	250
Kit Kat chunky	490	Cod batter -fried	240
Cream double	450	Scampi fried	240
Mars bar	440	Steak and Kidney pie	240
Cream crackers	435	Fish cake - fried	235
Duck fat & skin - roast	423	Lamb roast	218
Cheese cheddar	410	Chips thick cut - fried	230
Popcorn - salted	395	Bread white	216
Toffee bar	388	Bread wholemeal	216
Porridge oats	380	Beef mince - fried	205
Cornflakes	376	Salmon - fillets	200
Muesli - fruit & nut	360		
Bacon sandwich	358		
Chorizo	350		
Pork pies	328		
Garlic pizza bread	340		

The above table highlights the foods with the highest calories per 100 grams and most include processed foods with high carbohydrates, salt and sugar content.

Table 9: Calorie content of food types (low calorie) per 100 grams. [48]

MEDIUM to LOW Calories		Meals with LOW Calories	
Food type	**kcal**	**Food type**	**kcal**
Veal - fried	196	**Vegetables**	
Duck meat - roasted	195	Potatoes - baked	97
Beef roast	190	Onion - fried	95
Ice cream	190	Tomatoes - fried	87
Pork roast	180	Peas	76
Tuna - tinned	157	Peppers	33
Chicken - grilled	148	Cauliflower	28
Cream single	185	Carrots	27
Turkey - roasted	173	Leeks	26
Potatoes - roasted	160	Onion- boiled	25
Trout - grilled	150	Spinach	17
Pillai rice - takeaway	150	Cabbage	16
Pasta normal	140	Courgette	10
Rice white - boiled	130	Mushrooms - boiled	10
Eggs fried	120	**Fruits**	
Crab	115	Banana	80
Sweetcorn - boiled	110	Grapes	60
Ham - boiled	105	Satsuma	42
Haddock - grilled	105	Apple	42
Cod - grilled	105	Kiwi	42
Mushrooms - fried	105	Orange	36
Spaghetti	101	Peach	30

The above table highlights the foods with the least number of calories per 100 and most include whole foods (e.g. raw ingredients) with a better nutritional content. We can see that most of these foods are not man-made.

The golden rule is that if you want to improve your food choice habits, the quality of fuel entering your engine, then you need to select these low-calorie foods.

Food portion sizes

The food portions highlighted in the above table are per 100 grams. Your daily food portions will vary considerably, and it is difficult to determine the overall calorie content.

If you are regularly preparing meals with low calories per 100 grams (e.g. a serving of pasta, rice, or mashed potato), you may believe that you are eating healthily. The irony is that if you are 'loading' up your plates with 200 or 300 grams per serving then this will lead you to overeat and increase your calorie intake. In this case, you may just as well be eating food on the left side of the table, however, these may not be the healthiest options.

The table below highlights food portions that are larger, or smaller, than 100 grams that we typically serve.

Table 10: Typical food portion sizes for different foods [49]

TYPICAL FOOD PORTION SIZES					
Portions greater than 100 grams (3.5 oz)			Portions less than 100 grams (3.5 oz)		
Food type	Weight (grams)	kcal	Food type	Weight (grams)	kcal
Rice - white	160	215	Chocolate - Mars	58	240
Pasta -penne	150	247	Ham (1 slice)	30	32
Potato - mashed	355	247	Cheese average	25	110
Potatoes - roasted	155	250	Eggs average	60	90
Pork chop	200	514	Butter	5	37
BBQ ribs	400	568	Sausage	55	162
Steak portion (fried)	195	442	Crisps	34	100
Fish portion (fried)	130	298	Cornflakes	30	113
Hot chips (deep fried)	200	546	Peanuts	30	181
Vegtable soap	260	100	Bacon - fried	18	63

It should be noted that these foods are per serving. Once we include the add-ons to your meals then the calorie content can increase significantly. Having a portion of chicken (148 kcal) is acceptable on its own, however, adding a portion of roasted potatoes (250 kcal) increases the total calorie content to 398 calories.

Unless you weigh all your ingredients, the chances are you will have no idea of the total calorie content of most of your meals. As we seldom weigh our food portions, confirms the fact that most of us are not aware of our daily calorie consumption.

Control of our food portions

To control the portion sizes of our ingredients that we are cooking with, we need to understand the physical size. Most food portions now have nutritional information on their packaging, and they all refer to the calories per 100 grams sizes so that we can compare calories, carbohydrates, salts, etc.

Typically, a 100-gram portion of raw ingredient (e.g. butter, rice, pasta, potatoes), is equal to ½ cup, or one handful. For protein (e.g. meat, chicken, fish), a 100-gram portion is like the size of a deck of cards or the size of your palm.

The below illustration should give us a better idea of recommended food ingredient portion sizes.

Fig 7: Hand sizes for raw foods

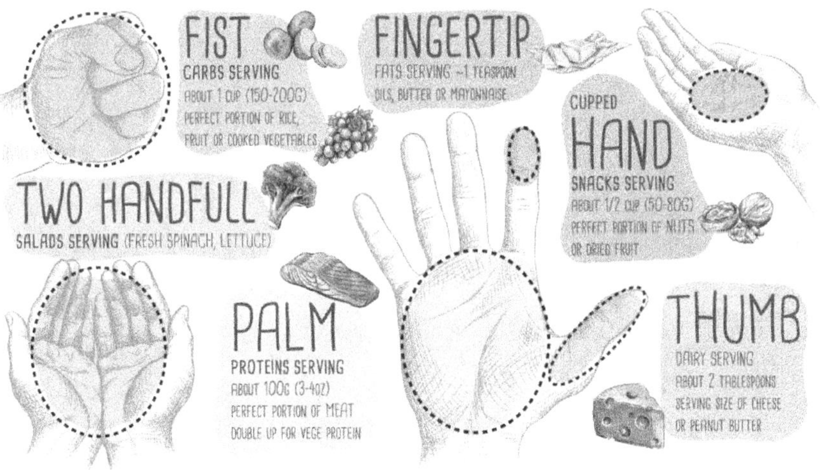

When we are preparing food and if we are not aware of portion sizes, it is advised that we consider weighing out the portions. A simple exercise, to get a good indication of size, is to weigh the food (e.g. pasta), then hold the portion in your hand (or cup). With time, you will quickly identify visually if a raw portion of food is greater than 100 grams, which will ensure that we are not preparing meals that are greater than we need. What is not on the plate, will not be a temptation to be eaten.

Reducing our food portion sizes, during the preparation, will help us reduce our food intake, our number of mouthfuls daily. These above facts highlight why we should all be on a mouthful (volume) reduction type diet as this is the most convenient method of reducing our food consumption and our calorie intake.

Summary:
- A sensible, balanced diet is the basis for healthy eating and wellbeing
- Always consider low-calorie, more nutritious foods
- Higher nutritional meals generally have fewer calories
- Some food portions have greater calorie content per 100 grams which will increase the overall calories contained in the meal
- When in supermarkets, avoid processed foods
- When in supermarkets, don't let sales promotions influence your food choices
- When preparing meals, we need to weigh our raw ingredients, so that we don't eat more than we should

15. REHAB OUR FOOD CHOICES IN RESTAURANTS (Step 5)

Third parties, such as restaurants, play a large role in our overeating. Their food portions are typically larger than what we normally eat at home. Furthermore, in most cases, we have no idea what the overall calorie content is, especially when we include add-ons, that we don't normally eat at home.

We usually associate a visit to a restaurant as a treat, or a 'feel good' moment that we had in the past. When our parents encouraged us to have a starter and then a dessert after our main course, this was another habit that we have adopted. Furthermore, they may have ordered more food than was needed, then we were encouraged to finish the rest.

At all times, when eating in a restaurant, we should always look for opportunities to reduce our overall consumption, the number of mouthfuls that we are having. If we are constantly challenging the rationale for having a big meal, this should help us make better food choices.

Our simple Rehab 'less is good' habit change strategy should help us avoid the temptation of a large meal, and is highlighted below:

…. *'why am I eating this large meal? Is it another habit of mine?'*

…. *'if I can't taste my food after 5 mouthfuls, why am I still eating this meal?'*

…. *'having a bigger food portion does not mean I am enjoying my food more'*

Below are several tips to help us reduce your daily food intake:

Reducing your mouthfuls in restaurants and takeaways

The calories and nutrition content of the restaurant, and takeaway, meals can vary substantially depending on the cooking method, add-ons, sauce topping and portion size. In most cases, it is almost impossible to calculate the exact calorie content as there are too many variables in the preparation and cooking process.

The table below should be a guide for the potential calorie content of an average meal that we have in a restaurant.

Table 11: Typical calorie content of restaurant food per serving [50]

CALORIE CONTENT OF RESTURANT FOOD per serving			
Traditional Pub meals		**Curries**	
Type	**kcal**	**Type**	**kcal**
Fish, chips & mushy peas	1268	Lamb Rogan Josh, rice	1010
Breaded Scampi & chips	1100	Chicken Korma, rice & naan	1078
Beef & Ale pie	800	Beef Madras, rice & naan	1175
Gammon steak, egg & chips	962	Vegetable curry, rice & naan	877
Chips - fried	423	Pilau rice	150
Full English breakfast	1531	Naan bread	200
Lasagne & salad	890	Garlic naan bread	255
Beef Chilli with rice	491	Poppadum & dips	377
Italian		**Chinese**	
Type	**kcal**	**Type**	**kcal**
Margareta pizza (12 inch)	1165	Beef Chow Mein	374
Pepperoni Pizza (12 inch)	1250	Sweet & Sour Pork	440
Spicy meat feast (12 inch)	1340	Crispy Shredded beef	525
Vegetarian pizza	775	Spare ribs	416
Cannelloni	760	Spring roll	169
Lasagne	780	Noddle's	282
Garlic, cheese bread	325	Special Fried rice (170 g)	269
Garlic bread - 1 slice	90	Prawn crackers (35 g)	200

The table highlights the fact that the calorie content of most restaurant meals is far greater than what we typically prepare at home, or a low-calorie 'ready meals' purchased from a supermarket. Furthermore, when in a restaurant, we typically have a starter and then a dessert with our main meal. When adding the extras (e.g. slices of breads, dips), this will further add to our total calories for the meal.

When we are eating out in a restaurant, we could be consuming half of our total daily allowance (2500 kcal for a man). More importantly, if we are counting mouthfuls, we could be having 40 to 60 mouthfuls at one sitting and this will harm our mouthful reduction target for the day.

When you have the option to order meals that come in different sizes, always ask for the smaller-sized portion. If you are already eating a smaller portion, then consider eating less of the add-ons such as chips or rice.

Removing our starter and dessert from your main meal will result in a further reduction in mouthfuls. In most cases, the main reason we entered the restaurant was for the main course.

Smaller food portions – examples

When in Indian restaurants, always eat only half of the main portion and reduce your add-ons such as rice portions, or naan bread. Consider taking home the leftovers. Compared to most meals, left-over curry is one of the nicest meals to have the following day.

Fig 8: Potential calorie saving if we reduced our curry portion by half

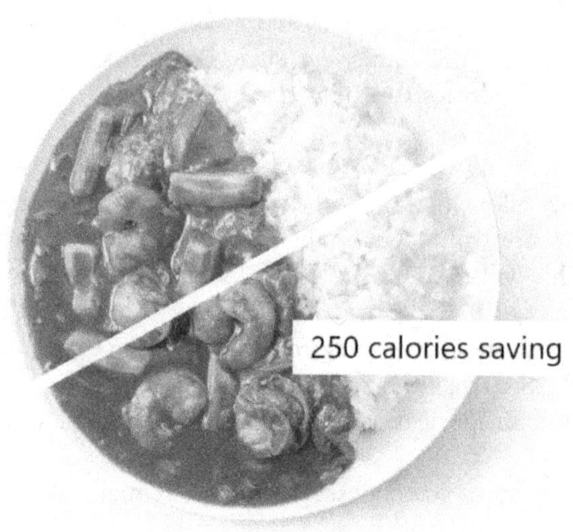

When in Italian restaurants, avoid or share the starters, especially the garlic bread with cheese. When presented with the main food portion, consider only eating half of your meal or removing a section of your pasta.

Fig 9: Potential calorie saving if we reduce our Italian portion by half

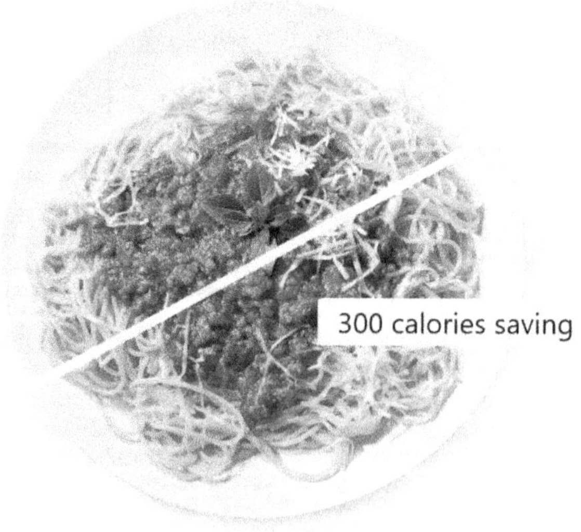

Pizzas are high in carbohydrates and fat content when compared to other meals of similar size. They usually come in two portion sizes, large and small. The larger 12-inch pizza size, with excessive add-on fillings (e.g. peperoni) can be as much as 1200 kcal, representing half of our daily recommended intake. Always consider ordering smaller-sized pizza portions or sharing the meal with your partner. One pepperoni pizza slice is around 150 kcal, so we should only have two to three slices, rather than a whole pizza, and consider taking home for a meal for the next day.

Fig 10: Potential calorie saving if we don't eat half of the pizza

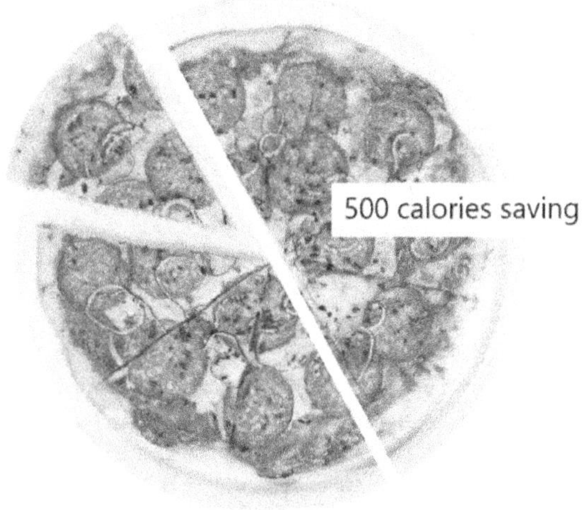

When in Chinese restaurants, consider reducing the add-ons, such as noodles and rice portions. Avoid, or share, the starters, especially the spring rolls and prawn crackers. When presented with a large food portion, consider only having half of the meal.

In the initial stages of the Rehab Weight Loss Plan, it will be a challenge for most of us to avoid the temptation to visit our favourite restaurant. If we are eating out regularly, and we are serious about losing weight, then it is highly recommended that we reduce or stop our trips to these restaurants as they can be detrimental to our good dieting intentions.

Once our 'less is good' habits are well-established, when we are finally in control of our eating habits, we could then consider re-visiting our local restaurants.

Desserts in restaurants

When in a restaurant, we believe that it is acceptable to have a dessert, even though we have just had a main course. In most cases, having a dessert has nothing to do with hunger. We are eating out of habit, first introduced to us when we were a child as a reward for our good behaviour at the table.

The issue is that most desserts are high in calories per 100 grams, having excessive levels of sugar, salt and butter content and are generally considered to be unhealthy food options. Furthermore, these desserts have limited nutritional value.

The typical calories per serving can be significant, depending on whether your choice is a high-calorie or low-calorie option.

Table 12: Typical calorie content of restaurant desserts per serving [51]

TYPICAL CALORIE CONTENT OF DESSERTS			
Popular deserts with high-calories		**Alternative low-calorie options**	
Type	kcal	Type	kcal
Apple pie (no cream)	429	Chocolate mouse	149
Banoffee pie	424	Ice cream (2 scoop)	166
Creme Brulee	333	Yogurt - Low fat	113
Lemon Meringue Pie	326	Sorbet (2 scoop)	104
Roulade	462	Jelly (sugar)	104
Sticky Toffee pudding	344	Supermarket Low-calorie	50-100
Chocolate cake	307	Grapes (228grms)	42
Carrot cake	374	Melon	22
Stilton cheese (50 grams)	206	Orange	62

The desserts on the left-side have a larger calorie content than the alternative low-calorie options. Typically, they contain the same number of mouthfuls, around five to six, however, the calorie content can be 200 to 300% greater.

If you are wanting to eat desserts at home, then most supermarkets now sell low-calorie dessert options (50 to 100 kcal) which you should consider as an alternative to the high-calorie ones. However, you need to appreciate that eating desserts on a regular, daily basis will sabotage your weight loss efforts and derail your diet.

In the Mediterranean, it is common to have freshly sliced orange, or melon, offered to you instead of a high-calorie dessert. Having had this dessert on several occasions, I find it a good alternative option as well as refreshing your palate.

Whilst on the Rehab Weight Loss Plan, or any other diet, to reduce the temptation, the 'what the hell, let's just do it', we need to consider avoiding all high-calorie desserts on the left-side of the table.

Alternatively, if you are wanting to eat desserts, it is recommended that you consider the following:

- Avoid all treats with high calorie per serving content, which includes desserts, cakes, cheese and ice-creams
- Substitute for low-calorie alternatives (50 to 100 grams per serving), such as yoghurt pots or fruit portions
- Alternatively, consider sharing your dessert with others

Sharing meals in restaurants

To help you reduce your overall mouthfuls for the day, there is no reason why you can't share a starter or a dessert. Typically, the main course was the attraction, the reason why we came into the restaurant in the first place.

Sharing a starter or a dessert will reduce your overall food intake by four to five mouthfuls. If you and your partner are both on the Rehab Weight Loss Plan, then this will be a good opportunity to help each other reduce your overall daily mouthfuls.

Restaurant meal leftovers

When eating in restaurants, we tend to finish our food portions as we have paid for it. For some, leaving food on the plate can be a difficult decision to make as it is a well-established habit. We need to re-think this habit, as this will be adding a further three to five mouthfuls to our overall total. If you are then helping your partner finish their plateful as well, this will add further mouthfuls to our overall total.

The cost of not eating the last portion of our meal only represents a small proportion of the total cost (e.g. labour, rent, utilities, etc) to produce the meal. So, we should not consider the cost of the leftovers, that we don't eat, an issue.

Once we start to regularly not finish our food portions, we will find that it is not a difficult decision to make. Asking for a 'takeaway bag' and having the rest of the meal the next day, will help make the decision easier for us and it will save us the cost of another meal. An alternative option would be to give your dog a treat, thus providing a good excuse to not finish your food portion on your plate.

Having taken your leftover meal home, it should not be another convenient snack to have between meals, or before bedtime. It should be an alternative meal to be consumed on another day. Too often these meals are considered an invisible snack and not monitored on any diet.

Summary:
- When in restaurants, always look for ways to reduce your food portion
- Consider sharing meals as this will reduce your overall mouthfuls
- Consider taking home the leftovers and having them the next day
- Avoid add-ons in restaurants as this will increase your total calories
- Having a desert has nothing to do with hunger, we are eating 'out of habit'
- Desserts typically have high calorie, sugar and salt content
- Avoid or reduce all consumption of treats (desserts, chocolates and biscuits)

16. REHAB OUR FOOD CHOICES IN FAST FOOD OUTLETS (Step 5)

Our trips to the fast food outlets are now habits that we have adopted along the way and play a large role in our overeating. Their food portions are typically larger than what we normally eat at home and we have no idea what the overall calorie content.

At all times, we should look for opportunities to reduce our overall consumption, the number of mouthfuls that we are having. If we are constantly challenging the rationale for having a big meal, this should help us make better food choices.

Burger meals

As previously highlighted, the size of our burger meals has increased significantly over the years, without us knowing about it. The table below highlights the typical calories per serving we could expect when ordering a burger meal.

Table 13: Typical calorie content of Burger meals per serving [52]

CALORIE CONTENT OF BURGER MEALS per serving			
Food items on their own	kcal	Meal (large chips)	kcal
BK Whopper burger only	566	Bacon triple cheese XL	1544
Big Mac burger only	522	Bacon double cheese	1352
Double Quarter pounder & cheese	723	Bacon cheese	1588
BK Double Whopper burger only	850	Big king XL	1425
BK Bacon Triple Cheese XL burger	1147	Big Mac meal	1350
Chicken burger only	487		
French Fries (small)	340		
French Fries (large)	680		

The calorie content of a standard single patty burger is around 500 to 600 kcal, which is like a packaged sandwich purchased from a high street outlet, or a ready meal from a supermarket. The issue is that when you order the larger burgers, the double and triple patty with extras (e.g. cheese and bacon), then your calories increase significantly. Then, when you include, as part of a 'meal deal', French fries and a sugary drink, your total calories significantly increase, and the overall content can increase to over 1000 kcal.

If you then decide to accept the offer to 'go large', with a large portion of fries (680 kcal), instead of a small portion (340 kcal), you are now increasing the overall calorie content to around 1600 kcal. In one meal you could be potentially eating 60 to 70% of your total recommended daily intake (2500 kcal).

Furthermore, their overhead advertising displays can be a temptation that some may find difficult to avoid. The latest burger meal offers a range of different sized burgers, from a single patty (638 kcal) to a three patty (1147 kcal) burger, whilst all appearing to be within a 20 to 25% difference in price and therefore are perceived to be a bargain. [53]

Instead of looking for the largest, most attractive burger, letting our 'more is good' habits from our childhood influence our choice, we should be looking for the smallest portion size, a single patty burger. Remember that after three to five mouthfuls we don't taste what we are eating so this should help us select the smaller option.

Most would agree that there is no obvious difference in taste between a single patty and a three-patty burger. If we were to select the smaller burger meal option, we will be consuming fewer calories and reducing the number of mouthfuls.

When they offer the 'go large' option, politely say no and this will reduce your mouthfuls and overall calories. Saying no to extra French fries and a large sugary drink will reduce your food consumption by around 20 to 30%. If you only eat a burger/sandwich on its own, this will further reduce your mouthfuls and calorie intake.

If the temptation to 'go large' is too tempting and you find it difficult to say no, then you should not visit these outlets, especially whilst on the initial stages of the Rehab Weight Loss Plan.

Other fast food outlets

Typically, there are two types of fast food outlets, one offering protein type meals such as fried chicken (KFC), beef (Taco Bell) and fish (Yo Sushi). The other, offering high sugar content meals, such as doughnuts (Dunkin Donut), chocolate muffins (Baskin Robbins) and ice-cream (Ben & Jerry's).

Some of these options may be perceived to be healthier than others (e.g. chicken or beef meals) as they contain protein. In most cases, when eating a single portion (e.g. a burrito) on its own, with a calorie content of around 500 to 600 calories, is acceptable. However, when we add extras such as French fries and sugary drinks, then the overall calories increase significantly. When visiting these outlets, we should always consider ordering the smallest option and limiting the add-ons.

The foods that have high sugar content, are typically eaten in-between our main meals, as in most cases, we see these as a treat. In most cases, these options can have excessive sugar, salt and dairy (e.g. butter) content and have minimal nutritional benefits. Our motivation to eat these meals has nothing to do with us being hungry. These meals are a well-established habit, a 'feel good' moment validated by your parents and constant advertising, via various media outlets, that confirm that they are okay to eat.

The main issue is that most of these meals don't come with any calorie information (e.g. an ice-cream serving). The table below highlights the fact that these items can have a high-calorie content.

Table 14: Typical calorie content in fast food [54]

<table>
<tr><td colspan="4" align="center">CALORIE CONTENT OF FAST FOODS per serving</td></tr>
<tr><td colspan="2" align="center">Protein type meals</td><td colspan="2" align="center">High-sugar type meals</td></tr>
<tr><td align="center">Type</td><td align="center">kcal</td><td align="center">Type</td><td align="center">kcal</td></tr>
<tr><td>KFC Chicken Tower burger</td><td>620</td><td>Wimpy Eskimo Waffle</td><td>691</td></tr>
<tr><td>KFC Chicken BBQ wrap</td><td>270</td><td>Cinnamon bun</td><td>426</td></tr>
<tr><td>KFC Mini breast fillets</td><td>125</td><td>Subway Chocolate muffin</td><td>394</td></tr>
<tr><td>Taco Bell Quesadilla beef</td><td>560</td><td>Cheese scone</td><td>350</td></tr>
<tr><td>Taco Bell Fajita Burrito beef</td><td>460</td><td>Custard slice</td><td>348</td></tr>
<tr><td>Taco Bell Nachos Supreme beef</td><td>790</td><td>Pink iced doughnut</td><td>285</td></tr>
<tr><td>Taco Bell Bean Taco</td><td>180</td><td>Baskin Robbins chocolate chip</td><td>270</td></tr>
<tr><td>Yo Sushi Tuna hand roll</td><td>132</td><td>Ice cream cone with flake</td><td>190</td></tr>
<tr><td>Yo Sushi Salmon & Avocado hand roll</td><td>132</td><td>Chocolate Iced ring doughnut</td><td>237</td></tr>
</table>

We can see from the above table that most of the protein-type meals, without French fries and soft drinks, have similar calories to a supermarket 'ready meal'.

However, the consumption of the high-sugar type meals, on the right side, should be considered as 'wasted' calories and should always be avoided, especially if we are on a weight loss plan. Consider opting for fruit or low-calorie yogurt portion instead.

Summary:
- When in fast food outlets, always look for ways to reduce your food portion size
- Consider sharing meals as this will reduce your overall mouthfuls
- Avoid add-ons (e.g. French fries) as this will increase your total calories
- When in local fast food burger outlets, say no when given the option to 'go-large'
- Having a 'treat' has nothing to do with hunger, we are eating out-of-habit
- Treats typically have high calorie, sugar and salt content

17. REHAB OUR FOOD CHOICES AT LUNCHTIME (Step 5)

For most of us, a quick, convenient sandwich at lunchtime is now a regular habit that we have almost every day, especially when at work. Sandwiches now come in all shapes and sizes and the added contents make these lunchtime meals attractive and irresistible. Our lunch-time sandwich meal can potentially represent 30 to 40% of our total food consumption, so we need to be mindful of our consumption.

Most sandwiches come in packaging and typically have their calorie and nutritional content highlighted on the pack. For some, the exact calorie content of the sandwich highlighted on the packaging can be difficult to understand. We need to be aware that we are wanting the total calorie content for the whole pack and not just for 100 grams only.

Eating large sandwiches at lunchtime, with all the additional fillings, can result in us eating excessive calories. Below is a table highlighting the calorie content per 100 grams, and the total for the pack, of the common sandwiches that we eat.

Table 15: Sandwich portion sizes vs calorie content [55]

SANDWICH PORTION SIZES / CALORIES			
Sandwich type	**kcal / 100 g**	**Grams in pack**	**kcal in pack**
Chicken salad	132	195	257
Ham and Cheese Panini	250	223	557
Salmon. Cucumber, Mayo sandwich	242	219	530
Tuna Mayo baguette	232	230	535
Ham and Cheese Toasted sandwich	268	160	429
Egg Mayo sandwich	156	160	253
Chicken Fajita Wrap	142	185	263
Triple Sandwch offers			
Bacon, Egg and Tomato Trio	304	256	778
Chicken, Ham and Prawn Trio	142	247	349

The table highlights the importance of checking the total calories for the whole pack of sandwiches, as they contain the 'real' calorie amount. We can see that certain sandwiches have higher calorie contents than others. The issue is that the total mouthfuls (5 to 7) will be roughly the same, however, the difference in calories could be significant. We should always consider having a low-calorie option.

A simple method of reducing our calorie consumption is to only have half a sandwich or share a portion with your partner. Or, consider moving the contents from one side of the sandwich to the other, and then not eat the one slice of bread. Or, consider having a wrap-type meal with the same ingredients instead. One, small tortilla type wrap is similar in calories to one slice of bread. Having a single wrap will potentially remove one slice of bread from our sandwich and should reduce your overall calorie content.

In recent years there has been a tendency from suppliers to sell triple-sandwich offers. Purchasing these offers can increase our number of mouthfuls and calorie content by 30 to 40%. A standard sandwich is just as nice as a triple one and we should avoid purchasing these options.

Sandwiches that are freshly prepared

Where sandwiches are freshly prepared, whilst you wait, the total calorie content is almost impossible to calculate. For some, there is always a temptation to add additional fillings to your sandwich to make it more attractive and appealing.

When ordering freshly prepared sandwiches we must be aware of the calories of the additional fillings as well as the add-ons that we may have (e.g. crisps or chocolate bar).

Table 16: Calorie content of add-on fillings in sandwiches [56]

SANDWICH MEAL ADD-ONS /PORTION					
Sandwich Meal Add-ons		Fillings / tablespoon		Sandwich Meal Add-ons	
Food type	kcal	Food type	kcal	Food type	kcal
Butter	112	Mayonnaise	94	Crisps - 1 packet	100
Margarine	110	Salad dressing	73	Portion of hot chips	560
Cheese - 1 slice	110	BBQ sauce	29	Chcolate - Mars	240
Bacon - 2 slices	250	Ketchup	19		
Egg - 1 portion	90	Mustard	7		
Meat / Chicken - 1 slice	6 to 10				

These add-ons should be avoided as they will increase our overall calorie total.

If we think it is necessary to complete our lunchtime meal with a packet of crisps, a bar of chocolate and a soft drink (non-diet), we will be adding additional mouthfuls, as well as another 300 to 400 calories onto the meal.

Summary:
- Lunch-time meals can represent 30 to 40% of your total food intake
- Avoid add-ons such as butter, mayo and salad dressing, or sauces, where possible
- Order low-calorie dressing or sauces if an option
- Avoid additional slices of cheese, meats, ham or chicken
- Avoid Triple-sandwich offers
- Choose salad options instead of large sandwiches

- Avoid add-ons such a portion of hot chips, a packet of crisps or chocolate bar
- Consider having a wrap with fillings rather than a sandwich

18. REHAB OUR SUGAR CONSUMPTION (Step 5)

For most, the consumption of non-alcohol (soft) drinks, and sweet treats (e.g. chocolate), are now well-establish habits that we have daily. These items are man-made, processed products, typically with high sugar content. Added sugar comes in various forms and includes; honey, syrups, molasses and sugar additives (e.g. sucrose), to name a few.

It is recommended that sugar in our daily diet, should not take up more than 5% of the total calories that we get from our food and drink intake. This works out to around 30 grams (two tablespoons) of added sugar per day. [57] Research shows that our daily sugar consumption is generally greater than it should be, especially our children who are ingesting around 52 grams more than their recommended daily allowance. [58]

Most of these habits were created in our childhood, as they were considered a treat, a reward for our good behaviour. Furthermore, excessive media advertising promoting 'good times', when consuming these products, also played a large part in creating these habits. The fact that a flavoured soft drink tasted nicer than a bottle of 'boring' water, with no taste, did not help our cause.

Having our daily soft drink, or sweet treat, is a well-established habit and is like smoking or taking drugs. The potential health warnings are either not fully understood or are conveniently avoided so we can have the next sugar 'fix', feeding our unhealthy habit.

Our consumption of soft drinks

It is a well-documented fact that most forms of soft drinks contain high levels of sugar which, in most cases, far exceed the daily recommended allowance and they are not good for our long-term health. [59] A can of cola (non-diet) can have as much as three tablespoons of sugar and suggests that we should not be consuming these products regularly. [60]

The average calories in a can of sugary drinks are around 130 to 150 kcal and, for a bottle, 170 to 190 kcal. [61] The issue is that we are consuming multiple helpings daily. If we are having five cans of sugary drinks every day, around 700 extra calories, on top of our main meals, then we need to remove these before we can start experiencing weight loss.

The table below highlights the calorie contents of a typical soft drink.

Table 17: Typical calorie for one soft drink portion [62]

CALORIES IN SOFT DRINKS			
Drink size	With sugar	Diet/lite option	Alternative option
Coke can (12 fl oz - 354 ml)	140 kcal	0 kcal	Conisder changing for water
Coke bottle (12 fl oz - 354 ml)	190 kcal	0 kcal	

Our consumption of sugary drinks needs to be treated the same as our food intake. If you are consuming a number of these drinks, on an average day, then you need to consider the extra calorie intake.

Whilst on the Rehab Weight Loss Plan consider avoiding all soft drinks, with high sugar content, or substituting these drinks for a Diet or Lite options that have zero calories.

Alternatively, consider drinking water which contains zero calories and is freely available, at no cost, from most taps. The health benefits have been well-researched and most of us don't consume enough water on an average day.

Our consumption of sweets

The issue, in most cases, is that we are having more than one sweet portion daily. For some, who are frequently eating sweets, when we add our total calorie content for the day, this will exceed our daily recommended sugar and calorie amounts.

A Mars chocolate bar can have as much as 33 grams of sugar which are almost that of the daily recommended intake of 37.5 grams for a man. [63] Having, say, three Mars bars per day (99 grams) represents around seven tablespoons of sugar. For most of us, we would not 'dream' of putting seven tablespoons of sugar into our cup of tea or coffee. This fact should be a simple motivating message to help us stop indulging in our unhealthy habits.

There is around 310 kcal per 100 grams of sugar. [64] Eating sweets, with excessive sugar content, will increase our overall calories for the day. Most of us don't consider this fact as there are only four or five mouthfuls in each portion.

The table below highlights the typical calorie content of certain sweets.

Table 18: Typical calorie content of sweets per serving [65]

TYPICAL CALORIE CONTENT OF SWEETS per serving					
Chocolate		**Biscuits, buns and muffins**		**Confectionary**	
Type	**kcal**	**Type**	**kcal**	**Type**	**kcal**
Cadbury Milk chocolate	259	Custard slice	348	Soft mints (100 grams)	375
Yorkie chocolate bar	301	Shortbread biscuit	396	Fruit pastilles (25 grams)	94
Nestle KitKat chunky	246	Chocolate chunk cookies	208	Fruit gums (25 grams)	80
Cadbury Crunchie	184	Caramel shortcake	340	Wine gums (27 grams)	87
Cadbury Crème Egg	177	Hot cross bun (50 grams)	156	Liquorice (26 grams)	91
Dairy milk caramel	225	Cinnamon bun	426	Marshmallows (30 grams)	98
Smarties	174	Blueberry muffin	366		

We can see that most sweets have a higher calorie per serving than most food types.

We constantly hear that when we are regularly eating processed foods containing high levels of sugar, this can become an addiction. There is no reason to doubt this fact as, in most cases, our consumption of these products has nothing to do with us being hungry. However, is it an addiction or a habit that we have adopted?

For example, if our mother packed a chocolate bar in our lunch box, then gave us pocket money to buy another one on the way home from school. Then, when we got home, there was a multi-pack of chocolate bars in the kitchen that we could conveniently access at any time, there is a good chance that we would develop a chocolate addiction for life.

Furthermore, if she told us that we were born with a 'sweet tooth', this will provide the justification that we needed to carry on eating our favourite treats, without experiencing any guilt.

However, if she had given us fruit portions instead, would we now have an addiction or a good fruit-eating habit? This fact confirms that most of our eating habits originate from our childhood and that they are not necessarily addictions.

Conclusion

If you have a 'sugar' habit, consuming an excessive amount of soft drinks and sweets daily, there is a good chance that you will never lose weight. We need to consider the extra calories that we are consuming, on-top of our three main meals.

For example; A typical chocolate bar (e.g. Mars) has around 240 kcal per serving. If we are having four portions per day, this works out to around 1000 kcal in total. Replacing these portions with four apples, or oranges, (128 kcal in total) represents a saving of 872 calories, an 87% saving in consumption.
If we are also having five soft drinks (non-diet) per day, around 700 kcal in total, replacing with water will save us 700 kcal, a 100% saving in calories.

Overall, we could be saving around 1500 calories per day. For anyone on a diet, this is a massive calorie saving and, by far, the easiest method of losing weight. As these options have nothing to do with the fact, we are hungry and have limited nutritional content, suggests that they are wasted calories that we must eliminate from our weight loss plan.

The underlying message should be that there is no such thing as 'healthy sugar' and they should be considered as 'wasted' calories. If we are regularly drinking soft drinks, eating sweets, biscuits, cakes etc, removing these items will result in an instant reduction in overall calories for the day.

Fig 11: A summary of 'Useful' foods that we should be eating daily

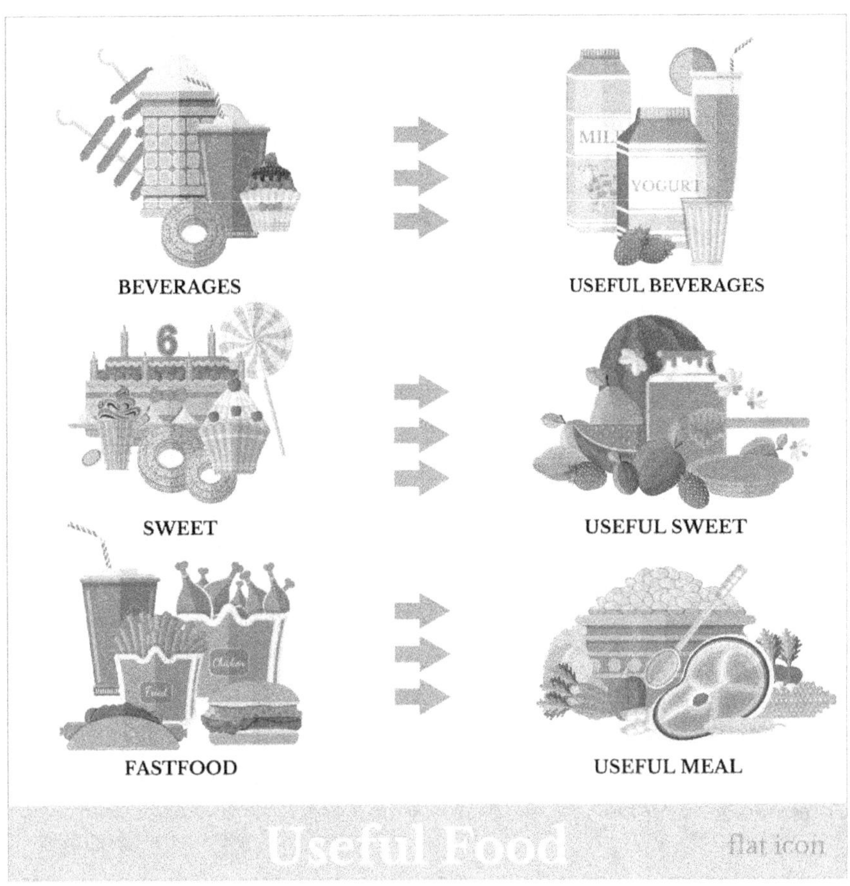

Summary:

- Most soft drinks (non-diet) contain excessive calories and sugar
- Any reduction in volume, or consumption, will result in reduced calories entering your body
- Unless there is a reduction in your consumption of these drinks, there is a good chance that you will not experience any weight loss
- We were designed to drink water
- Eating sweets has nothing to do with hunger, we are eating out-of-habit
- Sweets typically have high calorie and sugar content
- Avoid or reduce all consumption of sweets (chocolates and biscuits)

19. ALCOHOLIC AND COFFEE DRINKS (Step 5)

For most of us, drinking alcohol helps us relax and de-stress from the hectic lives that we live in. Generally, when we are enjoying these 'feel good' moments, the last thing we are wanting to consider is our drinking or eating consumption.

Excessive consumption of alcoholic drinks generally leads to us craving our favourite foods, which are typically high in carbohydrates, adding to an increase in our daily calories and overall mouthfuls. [65] Also, during this period, we may resort to drinking more soft drinks (e.g. Coke) than normal as we are craving a 'sugar fix' to help get rid of the after-effects.

If you are a 'heavy' drinker and on a diet, the chances are you will not lose weight, as you will be regularly consuming extra, wasted calories, which will be sabotaging your good efforts.

On the Rehab Weight Loss Plan, we are not suggesting that you stop drinking completely, however, we need to consider how much you are drinking at any one time. Your drinking needs to be treated the same as your food consumption and it must be in moderation. An overall reduction in the volume of your daily intake will result in fewer calories entering your engine.

Your subconscious mind and drinking alcohol

The fact that most alcoholic drinks are created from man-made chemicals, contain excessive carbohydrates and sugar content, suggests that we should not be consuming these products in the first place.

Our attitude to drinking alcohol is like our food habits and they were created in our subconscious mind and shaped by our upbringing and our 'feel good' moments. External influences, such as excessive media advertising, also played a significant part in this process, highlighting the message that it is okay for us to consume these products.

For example, if our parents were social drinkers, and they considered a relaxing moment, a meeting with friends, or a sports event, as a justifiable reason to have a few drinks, then there is a good possibility that you will do the same.

Consuming alcohol regularly is like a smoking habit. The process link is the same, seeing our parents, or peer groups, drink alcohol highlighted the fact that it was an acceptable indulgence, whilst excessive media advertising validated the confirmation.

It is worth considering that, as a child, if our parents had constantly highlighted the long-term health dangers of these habits, and we then repeatedly saw media advertisements showing people dying of liver failure or lung cancer, there is a good chance that we would not have adopted these habits.

There are several other reasons why we drink alcohol, which include boredom, loneliness and seeking friendship. These factors are not in the scope of this book as we are focusing on the reduction of our consumption, our mouthfuls, rather than the causes.

Reasons to reduce your consumption

Like our food habits, most of the time we are drinking in autopilot. For example, if on an average night you are having ten pints of beer, roughly 60 to 80 mouthfuls of beer, this will result in an excessive number of carbohydrates (calories) entering your body.

The question we need to ask is would 30 or 40 mouthfuls have been enough? As this has become a regular habit, we don't question the amount that we consume, and we tend to get forgetful, sometimes intentionally.

It is generally recommended that we should not drink more than 14 units of alcohol a week to keep our health risks low. This is the equivalent of six pints of average strength beer or seven glasses of wine, which works out to no more than two units per day. [67] Most doctors will confirm that one to two glasses of alcohol, in the evening, is acceptable for various health and psychological reasons.

Reducing your alcohol consumption has several advantages:

- Alcohol contains excess calories and any reduction in volume, or consumption, will result in weight loss
- Excessive consumption of alcohol may result in us eating foods high

in carbohydrates
- The after-effect of excessive alcohol consumption typically leads us to eat and have a larger breakfast than usual

If we are looking for a way to boost our weight loss plan, then we should consider reducing our overall alcohol consumption or change to low-calorie options.

How much are we drinking?

In most cases, we have never been told how much is enough, or counted how many mouthfuls of alcohol we are having at any one time. Furthermore, like our food consumption, we don't appreciate the number of calories that we consume in an average drinking session.

The table below highlights the potential calories when we are out drinking in an evening.

Table 19: Typical calorie content when drinking alcohol [68]

ALCHOHOL CONSUMPTION IN AN EVENING			
Type of drink	Estimated kcal	Glasses per evening	kcal per evening
Glass of wine (175ml)	150	5	750
Pint of beer (560ml)	180	5	900
Bottle of lager (330ml)	140	5	700
Single spirit with mixer (25ml)	60 +130	5	950
Glass of Champagne (125ml)	89	5	445

If we are regularly going out four nights a week and drinking five pints of beer, this would result in excessive calorie consumption of 3600 kcal per week, on top of your daily food intake. You will need to eliminate these extra calories before you can start to experience weight loss.

For most of us, trying to lose the calories from our food consumption is a challenge on its own. For some, adding another 3600 kcal will prove impossible, resulting in another excuse for a dieting failure.

How do we reduce our consumption?

The Rehab method of reducing our food intake, by reducing our number of mouthfuls, also applies to our alcohol consumption. We need to be constantly looking for opportunities to challenge the rationale for our consumption. Like our eating habits, we can change our alcohol drinking habits and we need to consider adopting the 'less is good' habit.

The first three to five mouthfuls of most drinks are always the most enjoyable. Our main underlying motivational message should be, if, after the first three to five mouthfuls we don't taste what we are drinking, then why are we still consuming the drink?

The most obvious method would be to eliminate all alcoholic consumption and not attend any social events. However, this is a certain recipe for failure, as almost every social event or family occasion, consists of having an alcoholic drink. This suggests that if we want to keep our friendships and our family happy, we still need to attend these social events.

The table below highlights examples of how we can reduce our mouthfuls for most of the common alcoholic drinks that we may regularly have.

Table 20: Typical calorie contents and alternative options for common alcoholic drinks [69]

ALTERNATIVE ALCOHOLIC DRINK OPTIONS					
Current Drinks			**Alternative Drinks Option**		
	kcal	Mouthfuls		kcal	Mouthfuls
TYPES OF BEERS					
Lagers - Draught pint (569 ml)					
Common lagers including Carlsberg, Forster's, Carling	130 - 180	8 to 10	Change for Half a pint (284 ml)	100 - 120	4 to 5
			Or change for common bottled beers (330ml) including Peroni, Budweiser, Corona	127 - 148	5 to 6
			Or change for 'Light' bottled beers (330ml) including Budweiser, Corona, Coors	88 - 99	5 to 6
			Or change to Low Alcohol bottled lagers	56	5 to 6
Ales (Bitter)- Draught pint (569 ml)					
Common Ales including John Smith's, Fuller's	203		Change for half a pint (284 ml)	100	4 to 5
Ciders and Stouts - Pints (569 ml)					
Common Ciders including Strongbow, Magners	190 - 240		Change for half a pint (284 ml)	100	4 to 5
Guinness	210		Change for half a pint (284 ml)	125	4 to 5
TYPES OF WINES					
White Wine - large glass (250ml)					
Common wines including Sauvignon Blanc, Chardonnay, Chardonnay	205	6 to 8	Change for smaller glass (125ml)	100	4 to 5
Red Wine - Large glass (250ml)					
Common wines including Shiraz, Merlot	210	6 to 8	Change for smaller glass (125 ml)	106	4 to 5
Sparkling wines (65 ml)					
Prosecco and various sparkling wines (glass)	80 - 90	4 to 5	No alternative and consider redoing number of glasses	80 - 90	4 to 5
TYPES OF SPIRITS					
Gin and tonic (210ml)	170	5 to 7	Gin and Slim line tonic (210ml)	115	5 to 7
Rum and coke (double)	168	5 to 7	Rum and Diet coke (single)	60	5 to 7
Brandy and coke	130	5 to 7	Brandy and Diet coke	55	5 to 7
Bacardi and coke	130	5 to 7	Bacardi and Diet coke	52	5 to 7
Vodka and mixer (double)	168	5 to 7	Vodka and mixer (single)	60	5 to 7

The drinks on the left-side have the greater calorie content and number of mouthfuls. The drinks on the right-side highlight the alternative options to help us reduce our consumption.

If you are drinking beer, the obvious solution is to reduce our overall consumption for the evening or drink less volume per drink. A simple option would be to change to a half-pint instead of a full-pint glass. Alternatively, consider changing to bottled beers which generally contain less volume. For wine drinkers, we need to reduce our overall consumption for the evening, or change for smaller glasses, if we have been drinking large glass portions.

When drinking 'hard spirits' with a 'mixer', we need to consider either reducing our overall consumption for the evening or substitute our high-calorie 'mixer' for 'zero-calorie' ones.

To reduce your alcohol consumption is not rocket science and all we need is some willpower. As we are not asking you to stop having a drink, only reduce the amount, this should not be a major sacrifice.

Recommended tips to help you reduce your alcohol consumption

- Consider reducing the overall numbers of mouthfuls for the evening
- Always order a smaller-sized beer drink such as a ½ pint or a bottle rather than a pint
- If drinking spirits with a mixer, always have a slimline or diet-version
- Miss a round of drinks. Although there may be peer pressure to keep up with friends, they will respect our wishes if we discuss this with them
- Drinking slower will result in a reduction in volume that we are consuming

If you are looking for further motivation to reduce your consumption, you should consider the following:

- Binge-drinking can be damaging to our long-term health
- Excessive drinking will increase your calorie intake and sabotage your weight loss plan
- Regular drinking of large amounts of alcohol can be costly
- Most alcoholic drinks have zero or limited nutritional content

Having an enjoyable drink in moderation with friends is acceptable, however, whilst on your weight loss plan consider reducing your consumption or leave out completely.

Let your desire for a healthier, happier life be the driver for reducing your alcohol consumption.

Our consumption of coffee drinks

In recent times, our consumption of coffee has increased significantly. Going back ten years, there was no coffee shop 'culture' and there were limited outlets such as Starbucks and Costa Coffee, to name but two. We are all now drinking more coffee than in the past, and we tend to visit these outlets out of habit, our 'feel good' treat, rather than necessity.

An interesting observation is how our visits to these coffee shops have now turned into an everyday habit. Previously, for most people, we had a cup of tea rather than a coffee. If your mother always woke you up with a cup of tea every morning, then, this habit extended into adulthood.

Now, on most days, we are having two to three cappuccinos and seldom have a cup of tea. We need to have our daily 'fix' and every time we walk past one of these coffee outlets, we are wanting to either order a takeaway or justify a reason (e.g. a meeting) for staying-in. As this coffee shop 'culture' was not around when we were children, it highlights the fact of how new habits can be created.

The issue is that for most of us, we are unaware of the calorie content, as they are not highlighted on the cup. If you are a frequent visitor, then you need to be aware of the calorie content of the coffees that you are consuming.

Table 21: Calorie content of coffee servings [70]

CALORIE CONTENT OF COFFEE TYPES per serving					
Coffee with HIGH Calories		**Coffee with MEDIUM Calories**		**Alternative LOW calories**	
Type - large	**kcal**	**Type - small**	**kcal**	**Type - small**	**kcal**
With milk		**With milk**		**No milk**	
Caramel hot chocolate	729	Caramel hot chocolate	343	Expresso (large)	11
Hot Chocolate	399	Hot Chocolate	167	Expresso (small)	6
Vanilla Latte	386	Caffe Mocha	163	Filter coffee (large)	4
Caffe Mocha	359	Vanilla Latte	143	Filter coffee (small)	2
Caffe Latte	298	Caffe Latte	108		
Cappuccino	253	Cappuccino	85		
Cafe Misto	169	Cafe Misto	64		
With Skimmed milk		**With Skimmed milk**		**With milk**	
Caramel hot chocolate	659	Caramel hot chocolate	313	Flat white coffee	108
Hot Chocolate	299	Hot Chocolate	137	Coffee (with milk)	18
Caffe Mocha	283	Caffe Mocha	137	Cup of tea (with milk)	18
Vanilla latte	257	Caffe Latte	60		
Caffe Latte	168	Vanilla latte	96		
Cappuccino	144	Cappuccino	49		
Cafe Misto	92	Cafe Misto	35		

We can see that the coffee types on the left-side have a greater calorie content than the alternative low-calorie options on the right. If you are regularly having three to five cups of coffee daily, you could potentially be adding another 500 to 1000 kcal to your daily total, without appreciating the fact. You could also be consuming 40 to 50% of your daily recommended calorie allowance, without eating any food of nutritional value.

If you are regularly visiting these coffee shops, then it is highly recommended that you order drinks that are less than 100 kcal, such as a basic filtered coffee or a flat white from the right side of the table. The options having excessive calorie content, such as the Vanilla or Caramel type drinks, should be avoided at all costs.

Whilst on the Rehab Weight Loss Plan, to reduce the temptation, the 'what the hell, let's just do it' moment, we need to consider reducing our visits or ordering low-calorie options only.

Summary:
- Most forms of alcoholic drinks contain excessive calories
- Excessive consumption of alcohol may result in us eating foods high in carbohydrates
- The first three to five mouthfuls of most drinks are always the most

enjoyable
- Any reduction in volume, or consumption, will result in reduced calories entering your body
- Some coffee types contain excessive calories and sugar
- Unless there is a reduction in your consumption of these drinks, there is a good chance that you will not experience any weight loss
- We were designed to drink water

20. EXERCISE AND WEIGHT LOSS

The old saying:

… 'if you want to lose weight you have to either eat less or exercise more'.

There may be some truth in this statement, as it is seldom that you will see a 'fat' long-distance marathon runner, nor will you see a 'chubby' cyclist participating in the 'Tour de France' bicycle race. The reason why these groups of people have lean body mass is that they partake in excessive exercise routines spending hours on the road.

The irony is that their daily food intakes are far greater than ours and they are still slim. For most of us, we have other more important things to do with our time and we can't spend two to three hours on the road, every day of the week.

It is a well-documented fact that any form of exercise is good for our overall wellbeing. It releases endorphins and serotonin in our brains and makes us feel good about ourselves. [71] Further benefits include lowering our blood pressure which reduces our risk of heart attack or strokes. Exercise also helps you sleep and is known to reduce hunger. [72]

Research has also shown that regular exercise does prolong life expectancy. [73] It is recommended that we aim to do some form of physical activity every day, at least 150 minutes a week (20 minutes per day) doing physical activities (e.g. walking, cycling, dancing). At least 75 minutes of this time should consist of vigorous exercise such as jogging, swimming, walking up-stairs, gym and team-sports. [74]

For those who are not participating in an active fitness programme, you should consider engaging in a plan to increase your physical activities. A fitness plan can include a range of activities, such as walking, running, swimming, going to a gym or partaking in a sport (e.g. tennis). A good activity to consider is dancing as it is both sociable and good exercise.

If you have never exercised before, or seen the inside of a gym, then we are not suggesting that you now go to the gym for one to two hours every day. If you have not been 'sporty' in the first place, I am not sure if it is a good idea to start a vigorous fitness plan.

Fitness covers a range of activities, so a short twenty-minute walk, or a swimming session, is just as good as an intense work-out in the gym. The most important factor is that you are enjoying what you are doing. If you enjoy what you are doing, then there should be no reason not to do it.

Any form of exercise is better than none. As the saying goes, 'Just do it', and this should be our motivational message, that is if we are using the same excuses again and again, to avoid physical activity.

Excessive exercise and food intake

Most people will say that excessive exercise makes us feel hungrier than normal. This is not factually correct as, in most cases, it is your subconscious mind 'telling' you that you must eat more as you have been exercising. This is a common misbelief and giving us a reason for another dieting failure.

If you are now doing more physical exercise than before and eating extra food as a result, this is not what you necessarily want. We don't need to supplement this loss of energy with extra food and it will be counter-productive, as you would be adding additional mouthfuls to your daily intake. As highlighted before, your body is an engine and no event, such as exercising, should influence the rationale for your food intake.

Furthermore, it is a known fact that strenuous exercise can make us put on weight. [75] If you are desperate to lose weight, you may not want to observe increases in your body weight when on the scales, especially when you are expecting to lose weight.

Our subconscious mind and exercise

Our attitude to keeping fit is like our food habits, created in our subconscious mind [76] and shaped by our parents, who may have not been keen on sport. If you had 'lazy' parents, there is a good chance that you may not have a favourable outlook to exercise. Also, our teachers may have asked us to do something that may not have been familiar to us. For some, who have never been correctly coached or shown how to play a sport, we will automatically have a negative attitude.

For example, my mother always believed that certain people were born musically gifted and the rest of us were not. She regularly told me, and others, that I was not musically talented, and that I could not dance or sing. I believed this misbelief for most of my life. Everyone now knows that playing a guitar consists of only three major chords, and, with regular practice, you will eventually be able to play one basic song. Also, we can all dance and sing, however, I do concede that some sound better than others.

In most cases our negative attitudes to exercise are linked to our past, perhaps family and friends constantly belittling us and making us aware of our inabilities and creating beliefs that we have had to live with for most of our life. We may have heard statements such as;

.... *'he is so lazy, he will never make the team'*

.... *'she is just not sporty'*

.... *'when he is running, he has the co-ordination of a galloping giraffe'*

There may be some truth in these statements, as some people appear to be more blessed than others and are good at sport. However, using these unhelpful statements to justify our failures as a child, is not fair and will live with us forever. Furthermore, they provide a suitable excuse for us not to participate in physical activity in adulthood.

For most of us, motivation and boredom are the biggest obstacles when it comes to going to the gym or taking a walk in the park. Changing our fitness habits isn't easy but once a habit has been changed, it will become a way of life and is easier for us to keep on track. We will have an appreciation that exercising our body has several positive benefits, especially if we start losing weight as a result.

A recommended method of changing our way of thinking is to question if there are any benefits to being unfit or unhealthy. If there are none, then this is a good starting point. We must improve our self-image to one that reflects who we want to be. We need to accept that we alone are responsible for making the effort to include regular exercise in our daily routine.

Excuses that sabotage our exercise habits

We can always think of reasons or excuses to not go to the gym but typically when we are there, we do enjoy the experience and it does give us a positive mental boost. These are excuses and if we are going to move forward, we need to acknowledge that this is what they are.

Partaking in an exercise activity makes us feel healthier, gives us a more positive outlook and we will feel more confident. Why would we want to sabotage these positive feelings by a negative statement that someone else has told us in the past? It is not fair to punish ourselves and we must accept that we are not perfect and move on.

If you are constantly making excuses to not visit a gym, or do any exercise, then you should consider going at a different time of day. Going to the gym first thing in the morning means that you have had no time to think about not going. Or consider going with a friend so you can both support each other. Furthermore, carrying out the physical activity for one hour only represents around 5% of your time in a typical day, so not being able to fit regular exercise into your daily schedule should not be one of our excuses.

Verbal repetition of a positive message

To make changes to your lifestyle, you need to constantly challenge your reasons (excuses) for not doing regular exercise. As previously highlighted, research has shown that using verbal repetition of a positive message can help re-programme your subconscious mind and change your habits for healthy ones.

If you are constantly using excuses to avoid exercising, then we suggest using the following positive statements:

…. *'no more excuses, I have loads of spare time in my life.'*

…. *'my body is an engine and exercise is good for it'*

…. *'doing regular exercise will give my weight loss a boost'*

Consider repeating these simple statements every time you are not wanting to exercise. With these statements, we are first highlighting the issue, the importance of exercising, and then providing a justifiable reason (e.g. our reward) for going ahead with our action.

By constantly challenging our rationale for not going, you will quickly see a change in your habits, and we will soon start feeling the benefits of regular exercise.

Typical calorie usage when exercising

We have all been told that most physical activities can help us lose weight as they 'burn off' the calories. Estimating the number of calories that we consume when exercising depends on several factors such as our weight, age, metabolism, duration, type and how vigorous the activity is. The below table should be used as a rough guide only.

For a 196 pounds (89kg) person exercising for 30-minute duration, the table below will give us a guide as to how many calories we could consume when exercising.

Table 22: Calories used during various types of exercise [77]

TYPICAL CALORIE CONSUMED WHEN EXERCISING			
Solo exercises	**kcal**	**Team sports**	**kcal**
Running (moderate)	369	Squash	533
Dancing	347	Football	356
Cycling (moderate)	333	Tennis	356
Aerobics	325	Basketball	289
Jogging	311	Badminton	245
Swimming (moderate)	267	Golf	213
Gardening	169	Bowls	133
Weight train (moderate)	156		
Walking	156		

It is worth noting that if we were to remove a chocolate bar (240 kcal) and a pint of beer (130 kcal) from our daily intake, it would be almost the same as running for one hour (369 kcal). Increasing our exercise activity has the potential to help us lose weight, however, if we leave out a meal (e.g. a snack), or reduce our overall mouthfuls for the day, this will have a bigger influence on our weight loss plan and it will certainly take a lot less effort.

Research shows that to lose 1.0 lbs (0.45 kg) in body weight we need to 'burn' around 3500 kcal. [78] If we were to exercise every day for a week, say jogging for 30 minutes (total of 2100 kcal), this suggests that we could potentially lose some weight if our food intake remains the same. Our exercise routine will have to be maintained for several weeks if we want to reduce our weight by any significant amount, say 10 to 15 pounds.

This will require discipline and a lot of effort, especially if we are not a 'sporty' type of person in the first place. Also, one episode of overeating, or consistently eating more than usual, as we are now exercising regularly, could derail our weight loss plan for the week.

Relying just on exercise, to help us lose weight, means we must vigorously exercise daily, and this is the main reason why long-distance runners and cyclists have a lean body mass. If we can't find the time, and effort, to put the hours into any exercise routine then we need to rely on reducing our daily mouthfuls as this is the easiest, most effective option.

Tips on how to improve your fitness level

For people who have never proactively participated in exercises of any type, and who are overweight, starting a fitness routine should be done with caution and in small steps. Try and identify opportunities to change your simple lifestyle habits, such as walking up the stairs rather than using the lift.
Consider walking to the shops, or cycling to work, rather than driving.

Increasing your daily physical activities will be easier than doing something that is not in your comfort zone (e.g. joining a gym). Small changes to your usual routines are easy to do and will ultimately lead to an acceptance that exercise is good for you as you will start feeling the positive benefits.

Besides your usual daily tasks, consider adding regular walks or other exercises such as swimming. The distance is not important, but you should aim to do the activity for at least 20 to 30 minutes. Going forward, we need to consider increasing this time to 45 to 60 minutes. With time, you will see the positive benefits of exercising which will motivate you to increase your current fitness activities to new levels.

If you find exercising by yourself is boring then consider team-type activities, such as playing tennis, football or dancing. We will find these activities more sociable and enjoyable, and with time, we will increase the duration that we are exercising, without us realising it.

For people who are currently on a regular fitness routine and are exercising at least three to five times a week, you need to consider increasing the frequency or the length of your workout, or activity. We can all do a bit more than we usually do and any increase in exercise will be of benefit.

If we can include regular exercise into our daily activities, this will certainly give our weight loss plans a boost. Furthermore, the benefits of regular exercise far outweigh doing nothing at all.

Summary:
- Any form of exercise will improve our overall wellbeing
- Regular exercise can help us lose weight
- Don't rely only on your exercise routine to lose weight
- Our subconscious mind plays an important part in our attitude to fitness
- Recognise that our well-established beliefs are the main reason for us not exercising
- Where possible, always look for opportunities to increase the duration of your fitness activities

21. REASONS FOR NO OBVIOUS WEIGHT LOSS

If we are regularly reducing our daily intake of food, the volume entering our mouths, by say 25%, from our original intake, there should be no logical reason why we should not start losing weight. More importantly, once we know what our baseline is and what our daily mouthful target is, we should be able to maintain our ideal weight and avoid the 'weight on, weight off, weight on' cycles.

If our body weight appears to be the same and the weight loss plan is not working, we need to review and consider the following:

- We have bypassed the stage one of the Rehab Weight Loss Plan, the rehab of our subconscious mind. We may have returned to our old 'more is good' habits of letting our subconscious mind dictate our food intake. Unless there is a disconnection between our thought process and our stomach, there is a good chance we will go back to our old habits.

- When calculating our baseline consumption, we have not counted all our mouthfuls during an average day. We may have forgotten to count the mouthfuls of our 'in-between' meals (snacks).

- We may have given up the weight loss plan too easily before seeing any reduction in our body weight. Typically, we should see a change in our habits, and weight loss, in two to three weeks. Our eating habits took us months, if not years, to create our present bodyweight. There are no short-cuts that we can take to speed up the weight loss process.

- The types of food we are eating, such as pizza or pies, are excessively high in calories or carbohydrates. Consider replacing these foods for options that have low-calorie content.

- During the week we are managing to reduce our mouthfuls, however, at the weekends we are overindulging and sabotaging our weight loss efforts. This is a common occurrence for most people as we tend to relax our eating habits, especially if there is sunny weather outside.

- Our excessive alcohol, coffee, or sugary drinks consumption could be disrupting our weight loss plan, as most of these helpings are high in calorie content. Consider substituting for low-calorie options or change for water. If we are not sure how much we are consuming at any one time, then we should consider recording our consumption (e.g. our mouthfuls).

- Our food consumption reduction targets are not aggressive enough. Reducing our mouthfuls by one to two mouthfuls a day will not help us lose weight and we are only fooling ourselves.

- We may be overindulging on too many snacks or treats, such as desserts, chocolate, biscuits and crisps. We may consider these a treat and they are not being counted. These treats have higher calories per 100 grams than other healthy options and are 'wasted' calories with limited nutritional content. Consider eliminating, or reducing, the consumption of these snack foods.

- Consider increasing your exercise activities. If you are constantly reducing your daily mouthfuls but appear to not be losing weight, then consider increasing your physical activities as this will 'kick-start' your weight loss.

- You may already be at optimum body weight, so you may find it is difficult to shed the last few pounds.

Finally, they say that perseverance is our best friend. Long-term weight loss is a marathon and not a sprint. This is not another diet that did not work. We will eventually lose weight when our new 'less is good' habit is well-established.

Regular monitoring of your weight

There is no greater motivational factor than looking at our weighing scales and discovering that we have lost a few pounds. Regular monitoring of our weight will give us a feeling of control and help us manage our weight loss plan. When we see that we have 'put on' a pound or two, we should then be able to identify when and where we have overindulged, or exceeded our mouthfuls, for that day.

Our weighing scales give us the feedback that we need when we are trying to lose weight and help us stay on a diet. There is a tendency to want to measure our weight daily to monitor our progress. However, our daily weight can fluctuate, depending on the density of our last meal (e.g. pasta vs a salad) and how much exercise we have had. We need to be aware that if we don't see a consistent decrease in weight every day, it does not mean that the diet is a failure.

We should rather weigh ourselves once every few days, or weekly, as this will average out any daily increases or decreases that we may have. If we are constantly referring to our scales, and we are not getting the result that we want (i.e. a loss in weight), this may provide us with another reason to fail on our diet.

Realistic weight loss targets

We need to be realistic about our weight loss targets, as research suggests that we can expect to lose 1.0 to 2.0 pound (0.5 to 1.0 kg) per week, [79] that is if we are constantly keeping our average calories below 2000 kcal for a man, and 1500 kcal for a woman, daily. If we have a weight loss target of, say 10 pounds, this should take us around 10 to 12 weeks. That is if we religiously keep on our weight loss plan. It may have taken us a few years, of constantly eating more than our recommended daily amount, to find ourselves overweight. This suggests that it will take us some time to remove the excess weight that we now have.

One of the main reasons why most diets fail is that to lose a significant amount of weight, we must constantly eat less for an extended period, say 20 to 30 weeks. During this time, there are numerous opportunities for our old habits to 'raise' their head, to derail our good dieting intentions, or have a 'what the hell, let's just do it' moment.

If the diet does not appear to be working, we then look for excuses to get back on our 'more is good' habits. In this scenario, it is not the diet that is at fault, it is our lack of will-power that is the issue.

If we have signed-up for the long-term, and we are regularly applying our new 'less is good' habit, we should naturally see a reduction in our overall body weight. This will ensure that we not only achieve our weight loss goals but also help us maintain our idea weight for good, without having to look at our scales.

22. FINAL THOUGHTS

When on holiday in the Mediterranean, such as in Spain, we will have noticed that the locals sit down to one to two-hour lunches on most days of the week and it is the highlight of their day. It is usually a very social affair with family and friends. In most restaurants, they have a 'the meal of the day' consisting of a three-course meal, with a bottle of wine, which is prepared on the day and at a reasonable cost.

The owner, or chef, visits the local food market in the morning to purchase the freshest ingredients for lunch. The food that is prepared is simple, innovative, tasty and the servings are average portion sizes. It is the highlight of my day, when on holiday, even though I have never been to the restaurant before and the menu is in a foreign language that I barely understand.

A typical 'meal of the day' consists of around 25 to 30 mouthfuls and proves that eating large food portions on our plate does not necessarily mean that we are enjoying our food more. The taste sensation is the main attraction, not the quantity. This shows that we can regularly sit down and eat a three-course meal and still not be overweight if this is done in moderation.

It is a well-known fact that they are generally healthy and live longer than most nationalities, so they must be doing something right. In the worldwide life expectancy league table, the Spanish have a life expectancy of 82.9 years and is expected to increase to 85.8 by 2040, the highest in the world. [80] They appreciate that the intake of food is the most important event in their daily lives and each meal should be a treat, a wonderful occasion.

Yet for most of us, our meals that we have three times a day, have become routine and now non-important events. We are not that concerned about the taste and the amount of food we are consuming at the time. For most, a quick sandwich and a bag of crisps, whilst on the run, is certainly not a highlight.

Most of our poor eating habits have been 'invisible' to us and we were not aware they existed. Now that you have read this book, you should appreciate the reason why you need to change these 'more is good' habits so they don't dictate our food intake. You now have the tools to start your 'rehab', the changing of your habits to 'less is good' ones. The importance of dissociating our subconscious mind from our stomach, by treating our bodies as an engine, will play a large part in how successful our weight loss plans turn out.

Having now re-programmed our eating habits and food choices, we will notice a difference in our awareness and intake. With time, having managed to successfully achieve and maintain our daily mouthful targets, we will start to experience a feeling of self-control. We are now managing our food intake and possibly for the first time in our lives.

When we have overindulged and exceeded our mouthfuls for a meal or day, we will start feeling the emotions associated with guilt and shame as we have let ourselves down. The good news is that we now have the 'playbook', to quickly self-correct and we can get back onto our diet, as we now know how much we have exceeded our food consumption baseline by.

Most of us are aware of the benefits of weight loss which includes lowering our blood pressure and reducing our risk of obesity-linked illnesses, such as heart attacks, some cancers and diabetes. This will reduce the risk of early death and is a potential cost-saving on long-term treatment. It is a 'no brainer', as they say, and a good motivating factor to consider if we are losing interest or wanting to go back to our 'old ways'.

Our simple, underlying positive, 'less is good' motivational messages should keep us on track:

.... *'why am I eating this large meal, is this another habit of mine?'*

.... *'after 3 to 5 mouthfuls, I don't taste my food, so why am I eating this meal?'*

.... *'having bigger food portions does not mean I am enjoying my food more'*

With any weight loss comes a 'feel good' factor, a new-found confidence that we can handle anything that life throws at us. We become re-energised and the joy and pleasure of eating will come back to us. Our new habits, which we will now have for life, will ensure that we achieve our weight loss goals and experience everlasting wellbeing, which is what we all want.

Good luck.

For more information and advice, then please visit:
www.rehab-weight-loss-plan.com

APPENDIX

MY TYPICAL DAILY FOOD INTAKE

I have been practising what I preach for over two years now and I have a completely different approach, or rationale, for eating food. The main difference is that I believe that smaller-sized meals are just as nice as larger-sized ones. By constantly challenging my rationale for eating and reducing the number of mouthfuls, a new life-changing habit was formed, and my 'less is good' food intake has now become second nature.

When presented with a large meal, I automatically think that I don't necessarily have to finish the meal. Food is now only a necessity and any treat temptations (fast food, chocolate, desserts), which previously I would have eaten without thinking about it, are not included in my thought process.

The meals that I consume during the day are now considered as 'top-up' meals and I typically aim for five to ten mouthfuls. On most days, my total mouthfuls are around 50 to 70, with an estimated calorie intake of 1300 to 1500 kcal, which is well below the daily recommended 2500 kcal. As my portion sizes are consistently less than what I usually have, I don't bother about counting calories or carbohydrate content. My new, 'less is good' eating habits mean I don't need to.

Most days, I only have two main meals, consisting of either a brunch or lunch, and my evening meal. Having a brunch, instead of breakfast or lunch, means that I am automatically reducing my meals from three to two, potentially a 30% reduction in mouthfuls and calories. This is now a well-established habit which I don't believe will ever be replaced.

I am still having, and enjoying, my regular 'go-to' (default) meals, consisting of Indian, Italian, Spanish and Chinese. The difference now is that my food portions are smaller in size and I avoid, or limit, the add-ons. When in a restaurant, I will always leave half a portion of rice or pasta, and only have one piece of garlic bread, or similar, if on offer.

My only sacrifice, if you want to call it that, is that there are certain foods I hardly ever eat, and these include: pizza, fish and chips, pies, bread, biscuits and cakes. I have no desire to indulge in these types of meals as my food choice habits have completely changed for new healthy types. If I was presented with one of these options, say a pizza, I would only have one or two slices.

I have substituted my chocolate addiction for oranges and satsumas, and I don't miss my daily sugar 'fix'. My consumption of sugary and alcoholic drinks is limited to the weekends and I seldom have more than two to three drinks at any one time. I am now only drinking to enjoy the moment rather than looking for an excuse to drink excessively. I still have a coffee habit however it is seldom that I have my favourite coffee type (cappuccino) which I have now replaced with a filtered coffee, which has also been a financial cost-saving.

I am not influenced by food offers in supermarkets, or trips to fast food outlets. If I went into a fast food outlet now, it would be to have the burger only, not the meal option. I have no interest in ordering French fries or a sugary drink.

In summary, the main point that I am making is that no personal or external factors ever influence my food intake. I only eat when it is a necessity and these new, good-eating habits and food choices will stay with me forever.

My reward

Over the course of ten to twelve weeks, I lost 15 lbs (7 kgs), and I am now at my target weight. This was all achieved whilst still eating my favourite foods that I previously had. Knowing that my new 'less is good' habits are now well-established; I don't need to ever look at another diet book or bother to get on the scales again. When I do overeat, or if I go away for the weekend, I now have the tools to self-correct and get back on track.

The table below will give you an idea of what I eat, and how much, on an average weekday, when working. These are my typical 'go-to' meals that I have on a regular basis. It should give you an idea of how many mouthfuls you could potentially reduce your daily intake by.

We should appreciate that everyone is of different size, height and physical build. The 50 to 70 mouthfuls per day may be adequate for me but for others they may require additional mouthfuls to avoid feeling hungry.

Table 23: My typical daily food intake

MY TYPICAL DAILY FOOD INTAKE		
Brunch meal	Mouthfuls	Estimated kcal
One banana on one slice of toast	4 to 5	150 to 200
One egg, one slice of bacon in a wrap	4 to 5	250 to 300
Scrambled egg (one) on toast	4 to 5	200 to 250
Yogurt pot with nuts / fruit	4 to 5	100 to 200
Cheese and Ham croissant	4 to 5	300 to 350
Lunchtime meal (if I had no brunch)		
Leftovers from previous night (small portion)	7 to 10	300 to 400
Lasagne (small portion)	7 to 10	400 to 500
Packaged wrap (i.e. chicken salad)	7 to 10	300 to 400
Packaged sandwich (i.e. tuna salad)	7 to 10	400 to 500
Salmon salad (small portion)	7 to 10	300 to 400
Supper meal		
Seafood pasta /risotto	10 to 12	400 to 500
Chicken curry with chapatti	10 to 12	400 to 500
Spaghetti Bolognese (small pasta portion)	10 to 12	400 to 500
Two pizza slices and salad	10 to 12	400 to 500
Other (snacks)		
Four / five portions of fruit	15 to 20	450 to 700
Nuts (three handfuls)	3 to 5	250 to 300
Beer (two bottles)	4 to 5	200 to 250
Total	**50 to 70**	**1300 to 1500**

Note: These are all estimated values and my mouthfuls are my target amounts.

INDEX

REFERENCES

1. Majority brits are on diet most of the time Huffington Post
    https://www.huffingtonpost.co.uk /2016/03/10/majority-brits-are-on-diet-most-
    of-the-time_n_9426086.html
2. Obesity and overweight World Health Organisation https://www.who.int/news-
    room/fact-sheets/detail/obesity-and-overweight
3. Global obesity rates expected to soar in next decade NHS UK
    https://nhs.uk/news/obesity/global-obesity-rates-expected-to-soar-in-next-
    decade/
4. Poor diet now killing more smoking NHS UK. https://www.nhs.uk/news/food-and-
    diet/poor-diet-now-killing-more-smoking/
5. Obesity and overweight World Health Organisation. https://www.who.int/news-
    room/fact-sheets/detail/obesity-and-overweight
6. 250 Million children worldwide forecast to be obese by 2030. The Guardian.
    https://www. theguardian.com/ society/2019/oct/250-million-children-worldwide-
    forecast-to-be-obese-by-2030
7. Treating obesity related illness will cost $1.2 tn a year from 2025. The Guardian.
    https://www. theguardian.com/society/2017/oct/10/treating-obesity-related-
    illness-will-cost-12tn-a-year-from-2025-experts-warn
8. Obesity-Related diseases among top three killers in most countries. The World
    Bank. https://www.worldbank.org/en /news/press-release/2020/02/05/obesity-
    related-diseases-among-top-three-killers-in-most-countries-world-bank-says
9. Global Poverty Facts World Vision. http://www.worldvision.org/sponsorship-news-
    stories/global-poverty-facts
10. List of countries by obesity rate Wikipedia.
    https://en.m.wikipedia.org/wiki/List_of_countries_by_obesity_rate
11. List of countries by obesity rate Wikipedia.
    https://en.m.wikipedia.org/wiki/List_of_countries_by_obesity_rate
12. Microsoft SmartArt 'Used with permission from Microsoft'.
13. A third of UK adults underestimate calorie intake BBC
    https://www.bbc.co.uk/news/amp/health-43112790
14. What causes food cravings Medical News Today.
    https://www.medicalnewstoday.com/ articles/318441
15. Unconscious mind Wikipedia https://en.m.wikipedia.org/wiki/
16. Unconscious mind Unconscious mind Wikipedia
    https://en.m.wikipedia.org/wiki/Unconscious_mind
17. Unconscious mind Wikipedia https://en.m.wikipedia.org/wiki/Unconscious_mind
18. Belief Wikipedia https://en.m.wikepedia.org/wiki/Belief
19. Habit. Wikipedia. https://en.m.wikipedia.org/wiki/Habit
20. List of fasts undertaken by Mahatma Gandhi. Wikipedia

https://en.m.wikipedia.org/wiki/List_of_fasts_undertaken_by _Mahatma Gandhi

21. What causes food cravings Medical News Today
https://www.medicalnewstoday.com/ articles/318441

22. Supermarket special offers contribute to obesity The Guardian
www://www.theguardian.com /society/2019/mar/27/supermarket-special-offers-contribute-to-obesity-says-report

23. Obesity growing portion sizes overeating The Guardian
https://www.theguardian.com /society/2015/sep/14/obesity-growing-portion-sizes-overeating-cambridge-university-study

24. A third of Americans dine out nightly at fast food restaurants Forbes
https://www.forbes. com/sites/garystern/2018/10/25/a-third-of-americans-dine-out-nightly-at-fast food-restaurants-a-nutritionist-speaks-out

25. Food delivery and takeaway market in the UK. Statisa Statistics & Facts
https://www.statisa.com/topics/4679/food-delivery-and-takeaway-market-in-the-united-kingdon-uk

26. More takeaways on high street despite anti-obesity push BBC
https://www.bbc.co.uk/news/amp/uk-45875294

27. Take-way clampdowns 'may combat obesity epidemic' BBC
https://www.bbc.co.uk/news/health-26546863

28. Fast food industry analysis 2018 cost trends Franchise Help.
https://www.franchisehelp.com /industry-reports/fast food-industry-analysis-2018-cost-trends/

29. McDonald's portion size change 1955 to now First We Feast.
https://www.firstwefeast.com /drink/2015/09/mcdonalds-portion-size-change-1955-to-now

30. McDonalds portion size change 1955 to now First We Feast
https://www.firstwefeast.com /drink/2015/09/mcdonalds-portion-size-change-1955-to-now

31. Television TV and TV advertisement influences children's eating
Encyclopaedia.http://www.child-encyclopedia.com/child-nutrition/according-experts/television-tv-and-tv-advertisement-influences-childrens-eating

32. 2018 World hunger and poverty fact and statistics World Hunger
https://www.worldhunger.org/ world-hunger-and-poverty-facts-and-statistics/

33. 5 Steps make affirmations work for you Psychology Today.
https://www.psychologytoday.com /gb/blog/the-wise-open-mind/201108/5-steps-make-affirmations-work-you

34. Re-programme your brain Wikipedia. https://www.wikihow.com/Re-programme -Your-Brain

35. Meditation Wikipedia. https://www.wikihow.org/Meditation

36. Addiction Wikipedia. https://www.wikihow.org/Addiction

37. Trauma is the root cause of addiction. Regina Leader-Post

Https://leaderpost.com/news/local-news/trauma-is-the-root-cause-of-addiction-according-to-dr-gabor-mate

38. Work out how much weight you need to lose NHS UK https://www.nhs.uk/live-well/healthy-weight/eat-well/cut-down-on-your-calories/

39. Is 100 bites the optimal amount of daily food. Advisory Board https://www.advisory.com/daily-briefing/2014/08/15/is-100-bites-the-optimal-amount-of-daily-food

40. How much weight do you need to lose? NHS https://www.nhs.uk/live-well/healthy-weight/work-out-how-much-weight-you-need-to-lose/

41. Food Menu JD Weatherspoon. https://www.jdwetherspoon.com/food/menu

42. Calories Checker NHS-UK https://www.nhs.uk/live-well/healthy-weight/calories-checker/

43. Why hot food more satisfying than cold How Stuff Works. https://recipes.howstuffworks.com/why-hot-food-more-satisfying-than-cold.htm

44. Eating slowly may help with weight loss Forbes. https://www.forbes.com/sites/alicewalton /2018/02/12/eating-slowly-and-mindfully-may-help-with-weight loss-study-finds/

45. Majority brits are on diet most of the time Huffington Post https://www.huffingtonpost.co.uk

46. Healthy diet Wikipedia. https://simple.m.wikipedia.org/wiki/Healthy_diet

47. Calories Checker NHS-UK https://www.nhs.uk/live-well/healthy-weight/calories-checker/

48. Calories Checker NHS-UK https://www.nhs.uk/live-well/healthy-weight/calories-checker/

49. Calories Checker NHS-UK https://www.nhs.uk/live-well/healthy-weight/calories-checker/

50. Calories Checker NHS-UK https://www.nhs.uk/live-well/healthy-weight/calories-checker/

51. Calories Checker NHS-UK https://www.nhs.uk/live-well/healthy-weight/calories-checker/

52. Burger King and McDonalds advertisements

53. Burger King and McDonalds advertisements

54. Calories Checker NHS-UK https://www.nhs.uk/live-well/healthy-weight/calories-checker/

55. Pret A Manger Menu Pret Manger https:// www.Pret.co.uk/en-gb/our-menu

56. Calories Checker NHS-UK https://www.nhs.uk/live-well/healthy-weight/calories-checker

57. Sugar: the facts NHS-UK https://www.nhs.uk/live-well/eat-well/how-does-sugar-in-our-diet-affect-our-health/

58. Children exceed recommended sugar level by 10 BBC. https://bbc.uk/news/amp/health-46720303

59. Most People UK are consuming almost 3 times recommended daily Diabetes Research and Wellness. https://www.drwf.org.uk/news-and-events/news/report-diet-finds-most-people-uk-are-consuming-almost-3-times-recommended-dailly

60. How much sugar in coke Coco-Cola website https://www.coca-colaproductfacts.com/en/faq/ sugar/how-much-sugar-in-coke/

61. Nutritional facts and ingredients Coca-Cola https://www.coca-cola.co.uk/brands/coca-cola-original-taste

62. Calories Checker NHS-UK https://www.nhs.uk/live-well/healthy-weight/calories-checker/

63. Mars (chocolate bar) Wikipedia https://www.en.m.wikipedia.org/wiki/Mars_(chocolate_bar)

64. New sugar limits can be breached by a bar of chocolate The Daily Telegraph https://www.telegraph .co.uk/news/health/news/10929296/New-sugar-limits-can-be-breached-by-a-bar-of-chocolate.html

65. Calories Checker NHS-UK https://www.nhs.uk/live-well/healthy-weight/calories-checker/

66. Why drinking alcohol leads to munchies The Independent. https://www.independent.co.uk/life-style/food-and-drink/eating-drinking-alcohol-munchies-why-drunk-food-study-a8861106.html

67. Alcohol Limits Unit Guidelines Drink Aware.https://www.drinkaware.co.uk/alcohol-facts/alcohol-drinks-units/alcohol-limits-unit-guidelines/

68. Alcohol Limits Unit Guidelines Drink Aware. https://www.drinkaware.co.uk/alcohol-facts/alcohol-drinks-units/alcohol-limits-unit-guidelines/

69. Alcohol Calorie Calculator World Cancer Research Fund. https://www.wcrf-uk.org/uk/here-help/health-tools/alcohol-calorie-calculator

70. Drinks menu Starbucks. https://www.starbucks/menu

71. Mental benefits of exercise NHS UK https://www.nhs.uk/conditions/stress-anxietydepression /mental- benefits-of-exercise/

72. Exercise for better sleep John Hopkins Medicine https://www.hopkinsmedicine.org/health/wellness-and-prevention/exercising-for-better-sleep

73. Even light physical exercise can help you live longer Time. https://time.com/5166564/physical-excerise-can-increase-lifespan/

74. Exercise NHS UK https://www.nhs.uk/live-well/exercise/

75. Gaining weight after working out, here's why Very well Fit https://www.verywellfit.com/i-just-started-exercising-why-am-i-gaining-weight-1231585

76. Motivation to exercise comes from subconscious mind Griffith University. https://www.news.griffith. edu.au/2019/09/18/motivation-to-exercise-comes-from-subconscious-mind-study

77. Exercise Calorie Counter www.wcrf-uk.org/uk/here-help/health-tools/exercise-calorie-calculator

78. Counting calories: Get back to weight loss basics. Mayo Clinic. www.mayoclinic.org/healthy-lifestyle/weight loss/in-depth/calories/art-20048065

79. Work out how much weight you need to lose NHS UK https://www.nhs.uk/live-well/healthy-weight/work-out-how-much-weight-you-need-to-lose/

80. Spain to beat Japan 2040 world life expectancy league table The Guardian. https://www. theguardian.com/ world/2018/oct/16/spain-to-beat-japan-2040-world-life-expectancy-league-table

ABOUT THE AUTHOR

Having tried every diet known to man, Shaun has always had an underlying belief that most diets don't deliver what they promise. In his opinion, to be successful on any diet requires 90% mental effort and 10% dieting application (e.g. eat low-carb meals). The problem with most modern diets is that they only concentrate on the dieting method and don't consider our well-established eating habits and beliefs inherited from our childhood.

He felt so strongly about this fact, that he decided to write a book about it called 'The Rehab Weight Loss Plan'. The simple 5-step weight loss plan will help you transform your eating habits for life without you ever having to go on another recognised diet again.

When not writing books, Shaun is a mechanical engineer specialising in the field of energy management and sustainability. His 'less is good' approach to life, not only applies to the environment, for which he has a lifelong passion, but also the promotion of social health and wellbeing.